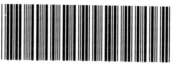

369 0280189

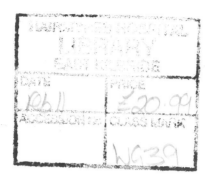

Cardiology: Churchill's Ready Reference

D1609992

For Elsevier

Commissioning Editor: Alison Taylor

Development Editor: Fiona Conn

Project Manager: Annie Victor

Designer: Stewart Larking

Illustration Manager: Bruce Hogarth

Illustrator: Robert Britton

Cardiology
Churchill's **Ready** Reference

Alexander R. Lyon MA, BM, BCh, MRCP PhD

Walport Clinical Lecturer and Specialist Registrar in Cardiology, Imperial College and Imperial College Healthcare NHS Trust, London, UK

Glyn Thomas MBBS, MRCP, PhD

Consultant Cardiologist and Electrophysiologist, Bristol Heart Institute, UK

Vanessa Cobb BSc, MBBS, MRCP

Specialist Registrar in Cardiology, The Heart Hospital, University College London Hospitals NHS Trust, London, UK

Jamil Mayet MBChB, MD, MBA, FESC, FACC, FRCP

Chief of Service, Cardiovascular Medicine, Imperial College Healthcare NHS Trust, London, UK

CHURCHILL LIVINGSTONE

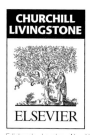

ELSEVIER

Edinburgh London New York Oxford Philadelphia St Louis Sydney Toronto 2011

CHURCHILL LIVINGSTONE

First published 2011

ISBN 978-0-443-06842-3

British Library Cataloguing in Publication Data
A catalogue record for this book is available from the British Library

Library of Congress Cataloging in Publication Data
A catalog record for this book is available from the Library of Congress

Notices

Knowledge and best practice in this field are constantly changing. As new research and experience broaden our understanding, changes in research methods, professional practices, or medical treatment may become necessary.

Practitioners and researchers must always rely on their own experience and knowledge in evaluating and using any information, methods, compounds, or experiments described herein. In using such information or methods they should be mindful of their own safety and the safety of others, including parties for whom they have a professional responsibility.

With respect to any drug or pharmaceutical products identified, readers are advised to check the most current information provided (i) on procedures featured or (ii) by the manufacturer of each product to be administered, to verify the recommended dose or formula, the method and duration of administration, and contraindications. It is the responsibility of practitioners, relying on their own experience and knowledge of their patients, to make diagnoses, to determine dosages and the best treatment for each individual patient, and to take all appropriate safety precautions.

To the fullest extent of the law, neither the Publisher nor the authors, contributors, or editors, assume any liability for any injury and/or damage to persons or property as a matter of products liability, negligence or otherwise, or from any use or operation of any methods, products, instructions, or ideas contained in the material herein.

your source for books,
journals and multimedia
in the health sciences

www.elsevierhealth.com

Working together to grow
libraries in developing countries

www.elsevier.com | www.bookaid.org | www.sabre.org

ELSEVIER   BOOK AID International   Sabre Foundation

The
Publisher's
policy is to use
**paper manufactured
from sustainable forests**

Printed in China

Contents

          Glyn Thomas

          Appendix 1 – Cardiac pharmacology   97
          Appendix 2 – Driving regulations and cardiac disease   104
          Appendix 3 – Bibliography   108

Preface

'To study the abnormal is the best way of understanding the normal'
William James, 1842–1910, American Psychologist

Management of patients in medical practice depends critically upon identification of abnormality, whether this be anatomical, physiological or biochemical. Knowledge of normality is therefore crucial, both to identify when disease is present, and to prevent overdiagnosis when it is not. This book is designed to provide a concise source of normal ranges for cardiovascular physiology and pathophysiology relevant to clinical cardiology practice in the first decades of the 21st century. In addition to covering routine investigations such as coronary angiography, two-dimensional echocardiography and electrocardiography, we have included many of the novel cardiac investigations now available, such as T wave alternans, intravascular coronary ultrasound and cardiac magnetic resonance imaging. This text provides the reader with normal ranges for a wide variety of cardiovascular tests at his or her fingertips, facilitating correct interpretation of clinical results. We hope this will be a useful reference text to the reader encountering patients with cardiovascular disease as part of his or her working life as a healthcare professional.

Defining normality is not straightforward, and in many situations abnormality is specified in terms of clinical significance for outliers from the normal range. For many parameters with a Gaussian distribution the normal range is defined as the range of values that ninety-five per cent of healthy individuals would fall within. The extrapolation of this is that five per cent of healthy individuals may have a value which lies in the 'abnormal' range, without any clinical significance attached to this outlying value.

A second issue is that there is frequently a grey zone of overlap between normality and clinically significant abnormality, and this reflects a continuous spectrum in the transition between the two states. For example, if the upper cutoff for systolic blood pressure is 140 mmHg, does the individual with a value of 141 mmHg have a diagnosis of hypertension with associated risk, whilst a second individual with a systolic blood pressure value of

139 mmHg has a label of normal blood pressure with low risk? Add dynamic temporal variation in parameters, and the potential for inaccuracy associated with all tests, and the scenario may become more complex.

Our message is that all clinical readings and measurements should always be placed in context, and clinical judgement is critical to extrapolate the findings of any investigation to diagnosis and treatment.

The authors would like to acknowledge the contribution of the late Philip Poole-Wilson, who was involved in the initial conception and design of this text, and whose teaching and influence have been a tremendous influence to all involved in research and care of patients with cardiovascular disease. We would also like to thank Dr Sanjay Prasad, Consultant Cardiologist at the Royal Brompton Hospital, London and Dr Vinit Sawhney, Clinical Fellow in Cardiology at St Bartholomew's Hospital, London for their valuable contributions in the preparation of this book.

AL, GT, VC and JM

TOPIC ❶

Coronary circulation

Topic Contents

Coronary blood flow

Oxygen consumption of myocardium at rest = 8–10 ml/min/100 g.

The heart receives ~5% of total cardiac output.

Myocardial oxygen extraction is high (~75%), and therefore there is little extraction reserve. Furthermore, the myocardium does not have great capacity for anaerobic glycolysis.

During exercise myocardial oxygen consumption can increase to > 40 ml/min/100 g.

Increased demand is met by increasing coronary blood flow.

Coronary blood flow is subject to autoregulation which is closely coupled to and driven by myocardial oxygen consumption (mVO_2). Autoregulation is lost when coronary perfusion pressure drops below 60 mmHg.

There is local metabolic control of coronary blood flow, thought to be largely mediated by adenosine and nitric oxide. There is additionally sympathetic innervation of alpha and beta adrenoceptors.

Coronary blood flow varies within the cardiac cycle and most flow occurs during diastole. During systole, extravascular compression reduces intramyocardial flow. The greatest resistance to perfusion is the subendocardial layer where the extravascular compressive forces are greatest and vascular pressure is reduced. Compressive forces are lower in the right ventricle and the drop in flow during systole is less pronounced.

Wave intensity analysis, using pressure- and flow-sensitive wires in human coronary arteries, has identified six predominant waves influencing phasic flow. It is postulated that a dominant backward-propagating 'suction' wave, generated by a fall in resistance of the coronary microvasculature with myocardial relaxation, is largely responsible for diastolic flow.

Coronary anatomy

Right coronary artery (RCA) (see Figure 1.1)

Arises from the right coronary sinus.

The first branch is the conus (infundibular) branch, which passes anteriorly to supply the right ventricular outflow tract. The conus branch may instead arise from the aorta.

In 55% of people, the proximal RCA gives off a small branch to the sinoatrial node. In 45% of cases it is supplied by the left circumflex vessel (LCx).

The RCA then passes along the right atrioventricular (AV) groove and gives off acute marginal branches to the free wall of the right ventricle.

At the crux (junction of AV groove and posterior interventricular sulcus) it supplies the inferior left ventricular (LV) wall.

The posterior descending branch supplies blood to the posterior third of the interventricular septum.

The posterolateral branch supplies the basal posterolateral LV wall.

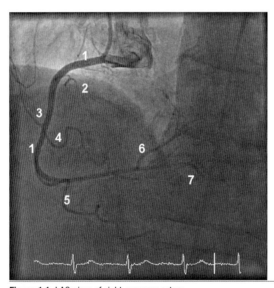

Figure 1.1 LAO view of right coronary artery.
1. Right coronary artery
2. Conus branch artery
3. Sinoatrial nodal artery
4. Right ventricular artery
5. Acute marginal artery
6. Posterolateral artery
7. Posterior descending artery

TOPIC 1 | Coronary circulation

Left coronary artery (see Figure 1.2)

Arises from the left coronary sinus as the left main stem and bifurcates into the left anterior descending artery (LAD) and circumflex artery.

The LAD passes along the anterior interventricular groove. It gives off septal branches to the anterior 2/3 of the interventricular septum and diagonal branches which supply the anterolateral free LV wall. Terminal branches supply the apex.

The circumflex passes in the left AV groove and supplies the lateral LV. It gives off branches to the left atrium and obtuse marginal branches to supply the posterolateral LV.

- In some cases the left main stem trifurcates into LAD, circumflex and ramus intermedius branches. The ramus intermedius arises between the other two. It supplies the anterior LV free wall.
- In some cases the left main stem is absent and the LAD and LCx arise from separate ostia in the left coronary sinus.
- In some cases the circumflex artery arises from the right coronary sinus.
- Left or right dominance: The dominant vessel supplies the AV node and gives off the posterior descending artery (PDA) which supplies the posterior third of the interventricular septum. The RCA is dominant in 85%, the LCx is dominant in 10% and codominance is present in 5%.

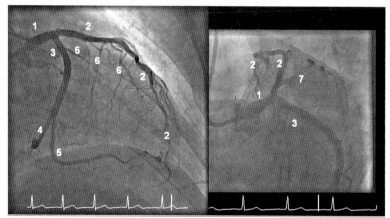

Figure 1.2 Left coronary artery anatomy. Left – RAO view, Right – LAO caudal ('spider') view.
1. Left main stem coronary artery
2. Left anterior descending coronary artery
3. Circumflex coronary artery
4. AV circumflex coronary artery
5. Obtuse marginal coronary arteries
6. Septal coronary arteries
7. Diagonal coronary artery

Coronary venous anatomy

Most venous drainage of the heart passes into the right atrium via the coronary sinus, the ostium of which lies in the posteroinferior interatrial septum. It receives blood from the middle cardiac vein (which runs in the posterior interventricular groove, alongside the posterior descending artery) and it is in continuity with the great cardiac vein (which runs parallel to the left circumflex artery). The anterior interventricular vein runs with the left anterior descending artery and drains into the great cardiac vein. The great cardiac vein also receives tributaries from the left marginal vein and left posterior vein. The small cardiac vein receives tributaries draining the right ventricle and also drains into the coronary sinus. The anterior cardiac vein returns blood separately to the right atrium and there are additional small veins that open directly into the cardiac chambers. The coronary venous anatomy when viewed in the LAO and RAO configurations is displayed in Figure 1.3.

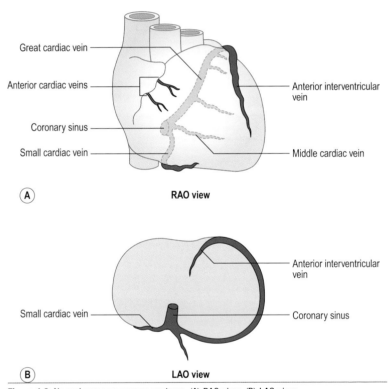

Figure 1.3 Normal coronary venous anatomy. (A) RAO view. (B) LAO view.

Coronary artery anomalies

Congenital coronary artery anomalies include:
1. Anomalous origin/course.
2. Intramyocardial (myocardial bridging). Part of the coronary artery takes an intramyocardial course.

3. Fistulae. The majority drain into the right heart (right atrium, coronary sinus, right ventricle, pulmonary artery).
4. Structural abnormalities. Stenosis, hypoplasia, atresia.
5. Duplications or single coronary vessel.

Clinically important anomalies

Anomalies associated with adverse events include:
1. Anomalous coronary artery from the opposite sinus (ACAOS). The coronary artery arises from the incorrect (contralateral) sinus of Valsalva with an anomalous course between the aorta and pulmonary trunk. Origin of the left main coronary artery from the right sinus of Valsalva with a course between the great arteries is associated with myocardial ischaemia and sudden death, particularly after exertion. Anomalous origin of the right coronary artery from the left sinus of Valsalva is also associated with myocardial ischaemia and sudden death. The mechanism is uncertain but may be related to abnormal vessel takeoff and direct compression by the aorta.
2. Anomalous left coronary artery origin from the pulmonary artery (ALCAPA). This usually presents in infancy with heart failure. Survival to adulthood requires adequate collateralisation from the right coronary circulation. Adults can present with angina, mitral regurgitation from papillary muscle ischaemia or occasionally sudden death.
3. Congenital structural abnormalities: stenosis/atresia/hypoplasia. May be present in early life with myocardial ischaemia or heart failure.
4. 'High takeoff' – The coronary artery arises from the aorta, above the sinotubular junction. Postulated association with myocardial ischaemia and sudden death.
5. Myocardial bridging – Uncertain pathophysiologic significance but has been linked to myocardial ischaemia and sudden death. Controversial.
6. Large coronary artery fistulae may cause a significant left-to-right shunt with volume overload and steal phenomenon.

Anomalies associated with congenital heart disease

Important coronary artery anomalies associated with congenital heart defects include:

Tetralogy of Fallot. The most commonly described anomaly is the LAD arising from the RCA and crossing the right ventricular outflow tract. This has important surgical implications as the vessel can be damaged during right ventriculotomy.

Transposition of the great arteries. Occasionally a coronary artery takes an intramural course within the wall of the aorta and can cause difficulties during the arterial switch procedure.

Pulmonary atresia with intact ventricular septum. There may be RV-coronary artery fistulous connections, coronary stenoses or interruption and coronary ectasia. In some patients, coronary supply is dependent on retrograde filling from the right ventricle.

❷ TOPIC

Evaluation of myocardial ischaemia

Topic Contents

Markers of myocardial injury and infarction

A universal classification system for myocardial infarction (MI) was published in 2007.

It defines five types of MI:

1. Spontaneous MI due to a primary coronary event, e.g. plaque erosion, rupture, fissuring or dissection.
2. MI secondary to ischaemia due to increased oxygen demand or decreased supply.
3. Sudden unexpected cardiac death with pathological evidence of coronary artery thrombus.
4. MI associated with coronary stenting.
   a. MI post percutaneous coronary intervention.
   b. MI secondary to coronary stent thrombosis.
5. MI associated with coronary artery bypass surgery.

Myocardial damage results in release of proteins into the circulation that can be detected with laboratory assays. These include troponins, myoglobin and CK-MB. Cardiac troponins are currently the preferred biomarkers as their detection in blood is highly specific and sensitive for myocardial damage.

CK-MB is an isoenzyme of creatine kinase, which is present in skeletal and myocardial muscle. An elevated level is usually detectable within 4–6 h of myocardial injury. Reference range is 0–5 ng/mL.

Cardiac troponins are myocardial contractile proteins. An increased value for cardiac troponin is defined as a measurement exceeding the 99th percentile of a normal reference population upper reference limit, measured with a coefficient of variation <10%.

Cardiac troponin T (cTnT) assays have a relatively consistent sensitivity with a cutoff (including 10% coefficient of variation) of 0.03 μg/L. The lowest level of detectability is 0.01 μg/L. cTnT is expressed by skeletal muscle in patients with chronic renal failure, and therefore cTnT measurements during acute presentations must be compared to baseline values in this patient cohort.

Cardiac troponin I (cTnI) assays are more variable and therefore reference to local laboratory assay ranges and coefficient of variation is appropriate. As a guide, a serum cTnI value of >0.5 ng/ml is evidence of acute myocardial injury with significant prognostic implications. Serum cTnI levels <0.01 are normal. cTnI values between 0.01–0.04 ng/ml may reflect myocyte necrosis, but depend on specific sensitivities and variability of the local assay. cTnI values between 0.04 and 0.5 ng/ml are suggestive of acute myocardial injury, and need to be placed in clinical context.

Troponin values may remain elevated for 7–14 days following the onset of infarction.

Myocardial injury and troponin elevation can occur without coronary artery disease. Examples include:
- Acute decompensated heart failure.
- Tachyarrhythmias.
- Myocarditis.
- Cardiac contusion.
- DC cardioversion.

Troponin levels may also be elevated in noncardiac conditions such as in acute pulmonary embolism, renal failure, sepsis and following brain injury or burns.

Myocardial territories supplied by coronary arteries (Figure 2.1)

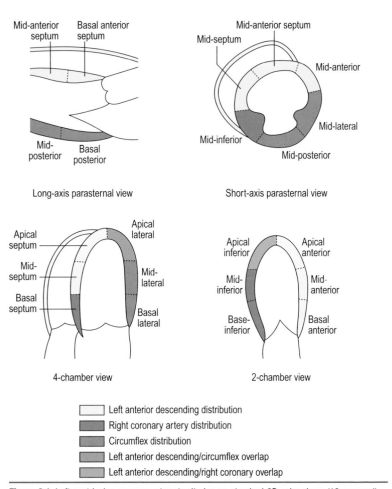

Figure 2.1 Left ventricular coronary artery territories on standard 2D echo views (16 segment).

The 17 segment model (see Figure 2.2)

Regional assessment of myocardial perfusion or wall motion (Figure 2.2)

- The left ventricle is divided into three sections (basal, mid, apical) in its short axis.
- The basal and mid segments are each divided into six segments.
- The apical segment is divided into four segments.
- The true apex (no cavity) is a single segment.

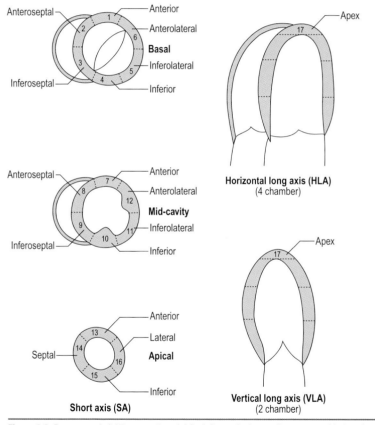

Figure 2.2 Recommended 17 segment model for left ventricular cardiac tomographic imaging.

Results can be placed into a polar plot as below (Figure 2.3).

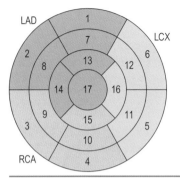

Figure 2.3 Polar plot display for the 17 segment model with coronary artery territory and recommended nomenclature.

Basal segments	Mid-cavity segments	Apical segments
1. basal anterior	7. mid anterior	13. apical anterior
2. basal anteroseptal	8. mid anteroseptal	14. apical septal
3. basal inferoseptal	9. mid inferoseptal	15. apical inferior
4. basal inferior	10. mid inferior	16. apical lateral
5. basal inferolateral	11. mid inferolateral	17. apex
6. basal anterolateral	12. mid anterolateral	

Stress tests

Stress protocols

Several modalities can be used to noninvasively assess coronary artery disease. Many techniques induce a form of cardiac stress to enhance detection of physiologically significant coronary artery disease, and therefore provide functional information which complements anatomic methods of assessment such as coronary angiography.This may be achieved with exercise (typically treadmill or bicycle) or by pharmacological methods or a combination of both.

Exercise ECG stress test

This test can provide diagnostic and prognostic information in patients with coronary artery disease.

Various standardized protocols are available. The Bruce Protocol is commonly used (Table 2.1).
- 3 minutes in each stage.
- Continuous ECG monitoring.
- Blood pressure assessment at each stage.

Target heart rate:
- 220-age.
- 85% target heart rate is deemed a satisfactory response.

Workload is measured by metabolic equivalents (METs) and reflects body oxygen consumption (VO_2). Resting VO_2 is approximately 3.5 ml/kg/min which is equivalent to 1 MET.

Table 2.1 Bruce exercise protocol with estimated metabolic equivalents			
Stage	Gradient (%)	mph	METs
1	10	1.7	4
2	12	2.5	6–7
3	14	3.4	8–9
4	16	4.2	15–16
5	18	5.0	21
6	20	5.5	
7	22	6.0	

Indicators of ischaemia:
- ST depression (planar or downsloping) $\geq$ 1mm relative to isoelectric line, 80 ms after the J point*.
- ST elevation.
- Increase in QRS voltage.
- Failure of BP to rise.
- Ventricular arrhythmias.

Advantages:
- Low cost.
- Widely available.

Limitations
- Lower sensitivity in comparison with other stress imaging techniques.
- Does not localise disease distribution.
- Interpretation is limited in a number of conditions including resting ST- abnormalities, left ventricular hypertrophy, paced rhythm.
- More false positives in women.

Nuclear imaging

Nuclear imaging techniques can be used for non-invasive assessment of coronary artery disease. Applications include perfusion assessment, viability assessment and measurement of left ventricular volume and function.

In these procedures, images are created from the emitted radiation of injected radiopharmaceuticals (radionuclides bound to marker molecules).

Single photon emission computed tomography (SPECT)

SPECT describes the use of a rotating gamma camera, which enables reconstruction to create a three dimensional image. Standard views are shown in Figure 2.4.

Radiopharmaceuticals in common use are: Thallium-201, Technetium-99m-sestamibi (cardiolite) and Technetium-99m-tetrofosmin (myoview).

After intravenous injection, the distribution of radiopharmaceutical represents regional blood flow. Distribution with stress and rest is then compared.

*J point is the junction of the S wave and ST segment.

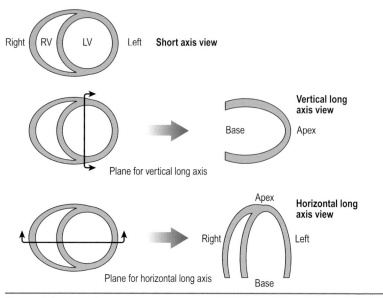

Figure 2.4 Standard left ventricular views in myocardial perfusion SPECT and PET. From: Society of Nuclear Medicine Procedure Guidelines Manual 2002 'Orientation for display of tomographic myocardial perfusion data'.

A perfusion defect that improves at rest indicates inducible ischaemia. A fixed perfusion defect represents infarction.

ECG-gated perfusion SPECT allows additional functional assessment including LV ejection fraction, wall thickening, wall motion and volumes. Technetium is more suited to gated SPECT than thallium.

Thallium-201 (201-Tl)

Potassium analogue. Believed to enter via the sodium–potassium pump of only viable cells and initial uptake is proportional to regional flow. Poorly perfused or infarcted tissue does not uptake up the tracer. However, tracer distribution in the myocardium changes over time and delayed imaging assesses its redistribution. Perfusion defects in ischaemic areas are filled in after approximately 4 hours. Resolution of the defect indicates viable myocardium. Detection of viable myocardium can be enhanced with delayed redistribution imaging or with thallium reinjection.

Planar images can be obtained before SPECT thallium to assess lung tracer uptake. High lung uptake is a marker of poor prognosis with an increased risk of cardiac mortality.

Technetium-99m (99m-Tc)

Sestamibi and tetrofosmin enter cells passively using negative membrane potential and bind to mitochondria within the cell. Unlike thallium, there is no significant redistribution, so separate rest and stress injections are required.

Higher-quality images are produced with technetium than thallium and radiation dose is lower. However, scatter problems can occur as the agent is eliminated by the liver. Tetrofosmin has less hepatic interference than sestamibi.

Pharmacological stress

Dipyridamole and adenosine are vasodilators which demonstrate areas of relative reduction in coronary flow reserve in regions perfused by stenosed coronary arteries.
- Unsuitable if caffeine/ theophylline taken in prior 12 hours.
- Risk of bronchospasm.
- Untoward symptoms include dyspnoea, chest discomfort, headache.

Dipyridamole: Synthetic. Inhibits reabsorption of adenosine and acts as an indirect vasodilator, increasing extracellular adenosine and leading to vascular smooth muscle relaxation. Standard dose 0.56 mg/kg over 4 minutes (up to 0.84 mg/kg). Much longer half life than adenosine. Effects can be reversed with theophylline. Avoid in patients with asthma.

Adenosine: Direct vasodilator. Very short half life. Infuse at 140 μg/kg/minute for 6 minutes. Stimulates A1 purine receptors in SA node and AV node and can cause conduction disturbance.

Positron emission tomography

This radionuclide imaging technique can be applied to the assessment of myocardial perfusion and viability.

The tracers used in this modality emit positrons when they decay. Positrons and electrons collide to form two high-energy photons which move in opposite directions. Paired detectors register the coincident arrival of photon pairs, and from this an image is reconstructed.
- For perfusion assessment a pharmacological stress agent is such as adenosine or dobutamine is required. The perfusion tracer is commonly 13N-ammonia or rubidium-82.
- For viability assessment, a metabolic tracer is used. This is commonly FDG (18-fluorodeoxyglucose). FDG is a glucose analogue which detects metabolic activity. Viability is indicated by areas of myocardium demonstrating reduced blood flow but remaining metabolically active.
- PET has better spatial resolution than SPECT and attenuation problems are less likely.
- Applications include assessment in obese patients and multivessel disease.
- PET is limited by the need for either an on site cyclotron or generator and is not as widely available as SPECT.

Stress echocardiography

- This modality involves transthoracic echocardiographic assessment at rest and with stress. Stress induced regional wall motion changes are then assessed.
- Exercise or pharmacological stress can be used.

Disadvantages of exercise: 90 second time window after peak exercise for optimum sensitivity. Increased ventilation/respiratory excursion makes image acquisition more difficult.

Typical pharmacological agents: dobutamine (+/− atropine), adenosine, dipyridamole.

Dobutamine effects: Increased contractility and heart rate, reduced systemic vascular resistance; possible side effects: palpitations, flushing, arrhythmias, drop in blood pressure.

The dobutamine dose is 5–10 μg/kg/min increased in increments to max 40 μg/kg/min.

Atropine can be given in addition to increase heart rate to target.

Views:
- Parasternal: Short axis.
- Apical: 4 chamber, 2 chamber and 3 chamber.

A number can be assigned to each segment and a wall motion score can be calculated:
1. Normal.
2. Hypokinesis.

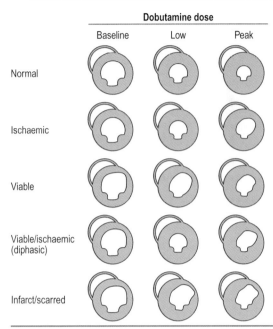

Figure 2.5 Short axis view of left ventricle at end systole demonstrating various responses of the anterolateral wall to low and high doses of dobutamine infusion.

3. Akinesis.
4. Dyskinesis.
5. Aneurysmal.

Interpretation: (Figure 2.5)
- Normal contractility at baseline and low dose but abnormal at peak dose = ischaemia.
- Abnormal at rest but improving contractility at low and peak dose = stunned.
- Abnormal at rest, improving at low dose, sustained improvement at high dose = viable and non-ischaemic
- Abnormal at rest, improving at low dose and deteriorating at peak dose (biphasic) = viable and ischaemic
- Abnormal at rest, low dose and high dose = scarred.
  Advantages: No ionising radiation
  Limitations: Need for operator expertise, echo windows may be poor

Cardiac magnetic resonance imaging (see Figure 2.6)

Magnetic resonance imaging (MRI) involves the application of a strong magnetic field to the body. Radio wave energy is then applied to the area of interest. The resulting signal is then processed to generate an image.

Techniques used in the assessment of coronary artery disease include the following:
- Assessment of resting ventricular function, wall thickness and regional wall motion

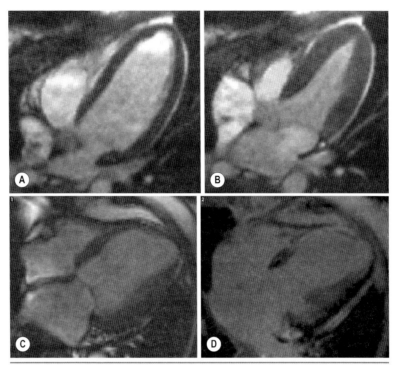

Figure 2.6 Cardiac magnetic resonance imaging. Four-chamber cine images of a normal heart at end diastole (A) and end systole (B). Equivalent end-diastolic views of a heart demonstrating chronic distal septal and apical myocardial infarction at baseline (C) and after late gadolinium enhancement (D).

- Dobutamine stress MRI can be performed using standard protocols. Regional wall motion changes in 17 segments are analysed as for stress echocardiography.
- Myocardial perfusion MRI can be performed using standard protocols. Myocardial perfusion at rest and with adenosine is assessed by measuring first pass signals after a bolus injection of gadolinium contrast. Hypoperfused areas have reduced signal intensity and invariably involve the subendocardium if ischaemia is present.
- Delayed imaging using gadolinium allows direct identification of necrosis or scar. Gadolinium contrast distribution is limited to the extracellular space and is retained preferentially both in necrotic tissue and in scarred myocardium. An enhancement study performed 10 minutes after contrast injection assesses contrast elimination. Late gadolinium enhancement (LGE) refers to retention of gadolinium, which appears as a bright signal.

Late gadolinium enhancement can be used to assess viability. Impaired contractility without wall thinning and without late enhancement indicates hibernating viable myocardium. Recovery of function with revascularisation can be predicted by the transmural extent of scarring. Transmural enhancement percentage is inversely related to the likelihood of functional recovery.

Advantages include:
- No ionising radiation.
- Large field of view.
- Good spatial and temporal resolution.

Limitations include incompatibility with ferromagnetic substances and patient tolerance due to claustrophobia. Resolution of magnetic resonance coronary angiography is not sufficient to replace traditional methods of anatomic assessment.

Coronary calcification imaging

Coronary calcification imaging may be used as a non-invasive surrogate marker of overall coronary artery disease burden.

Coronary artery calcification occurs almost exclusively in atherosclerosis. Detection of calcium with CT is used to assess plaque burden. This has been translated into a calcium score: Agatston score (Table 2.2). The score is generated from the product of calcium plaque area and calcium plaque density (Hounsfield number).

Table 2.2 **Description of plaque burden according to calcium score**	
0	No identifiable atherosclerotic plaque
1–10	Minimal plaque burden
11–100	Mild plaque burden
101–400	Moderate plaque burden
Over 400	Extensive plaque burden

The absolute value can also be matched against expected score for age.

Electron beam CT (EBCT) has a rapid scan speed to reduce motion artefact. Multidetector CT scanning (MDCT) can also be used but acquisition times are longer and radiation dose is higher.
- Not all plaque contains calcium and calcium is not a marker for vulnerable plaque.
- There is evidence that calcium scoring can predict risk of future coronary events but there is no evidence that screening improves outcome.

Possible applications:
- Screening of asymptomatic patients with intermediate risk.
- Assessment of patients with atypical symptoms.

Diagnostic adjuncts in angiography and percutaneous intervention

There are now technologies in common use that provide important supplementary information during invasive coronary angiography and can therefore aid decision making.

Pressure wire

The pressure wire study allows physiological assessment of coronary lesions (Figure 2.7).

The test result is expressed as fractional flow reserve (FFR). It is defined as the ratio of maximum blood flow in the presence of a stenosis, divided by maximum blood flow in the absence of a stenosis. It is the ratio of two measured pressures: coronary pressure distal to the stenosis (Pd) divided by aortic pressure (Pa), under conditions of maximal hyperaemia.

- The discriminant value for a functionally flow-limiting significant lesion is <0.75.
- The FFR of a non-flow-limiting lesion is > 0.80.
- FFR 0.75-0.80 represents an intermediate 'grey' zone.

Applications include:
- Assessment of angiographically intermediate lesions.
- Where non-invasive myocardial perfusion data are unavailable.
- Assessment in multivessel disease.

Disadvantages include:
- May cause vessel injury.
- Complications associated with adenosine.
- Sources of confounding include submaximal hyperaemia, microvascular disease, left ventricular hypertrophy and the presence of serial stenoses.

Procedure
- 0.014 inch pressure wire passed through guide catheter
- Calibrated against guide catheter transduced pressure
- Passed through lesion
- Maximal hyperaemia induced
- Wire pulled back across lesion with continuous guide catheter and sensor pressure recording

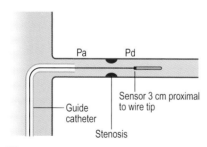

$$FFR = \frac{Pd}{Pa}$$

FFR is measured in state of hyperaemia. Adenosine dilates the distal microvasculature. Pressure falls distal to the lesion

Adenosine administration;
IV – 140 μg/kg
IC bolus – for RCA 12 μg/for LAD 18 μg

Figure 2.7 Schematic of fractional flow reserve (FFR) measurement in a coronary artery.

Intravascular ultrasound

Intravascular ultrasound (IVUS) allows coronary artery visualisation during cardiac catheterisation and provides high resolution images of the vessel lumen and wall.

A flexible ultrasound probe is passed through the angiographic catheter into the vessel of interest. It is then pulled proximally, usually with the use of a motorised attachment at a fixed speed, whilst images are obtained in real time.

This modality allows assessment of vessel dimensions and morphology, lesion composition and length.

Applications include:
- Evaluation of left main stem disease, ostial stenoses, complex lesions and other areas of interest not well visualized on angiography.
- Assessment of stent expansion or restenosis.

Disadvantages:
- May cause vessel injury or spasm.
- For vessels >1.5 mm.
- Increases length of procedure.

TOPIC ❸

Preventative cardiology

Topic Contents

Smoking

Smoking independently increases cardiovascular risk 2–4-fold compared with non-smokers and combines with other risk factors to greatly increase cardiovascular risk.

Relative risk reduction of smoking cessation falls to match that of a life-long non-smoker after 10–15 years.

Obesity and diet

Body mass index (BMI) = body weight (kg)/height (m)

World Health Organization (WHO)/National Institute of Health (NIH) Classification

BMI 25 – 29.9 kg/m^2 = overweight

BMI $\geq$ 30 kg/m^2 = obese

Waist circumference

Waist circumference = circumference (cm) between lower rib and anterior-superior iliac spine

World Health Organization (WHO)/National Heart Lung and Blood Institute (NHLBI) Classification

WC $\geq$ 94 cm (M)/80 cm (F) = no more weight should be gained

WC $\geq$ 102 cm (M)/88 cm (F) = advise weight reduction

Hypertension

European Society of Hypertension (ESH)/European Society of Cardiology (ESC) Classification, 2007

See Table 3.1.

Table 3.1 **European Society of Hypertension (ESH)/European Society of Cardiology (ESC) Classification**

Category	Systolic (mmHg)		Diastolic (mmHg)
Optimal	< 120	and	< 80
Normal	120–129	and/or	80–85
High normal	130–139	and/or	86–89
Grade 1 hypertension	140–159	and/or	90–99
Grade 2 hypertension	160–179	and/or	100–109
Grade 3 hypertension	$\geq$ 180	and/or	$\geq$ 110
Isolated systolic hypertension	$\geq$ 140	and	<90

Recommended daily salt intake

< 3.8 g/day (equivalent to sodium intake of 65 mmol/day)

Hypercholesterolaemia

ESC Guidelines

See Table 3.2.

Table 3.2 **European Society of Cardiology (ESC) Classification of Hypercholesterolaemia**

Category	Total cholesterol (mmol/L)	LDL (mmol/L)
General population	<5 (190 mg/dl)	< 3 (115 mg/dl)
High risk	< 4 (155 mg/dl)	< 2 (80 mg/dl)

Diabetes and metabolic syndrome

ESC Guidelines on treatment targets in type 2 diabetes

See Table 3.3.

Table 3.3 European Society of Cardiology (ESC) Guidelines on treatment targets in type 2 diabetes		
Category	Unit	Target
HbA$_{1c}$	HbA$_{1c}$ (%)	$\leq$ 6.5
Plasma glucose	Fasting/pre-prandial mmol/L (mg/dl)	< 6.0 (110)
Blood pressure	mmHg	$\leq$ 130/80
Total cholesterol	mmol/L (mg/dl)	< 4 (155)
LDL cholesterol	mmol/L (mg/dl)	< 2 80

International Diabetes Federation (IDF) definition of metabolic syndrome

Metabolic syndrome is a combination of cardiovascular risk factors in individuals with obesity or insulin resistance (specifically, central obesity, hypertension, low HDL cholesterol, raised triglycerides and hyperglycaemia).

Must have:
1. Central obesity (defined by ethnic-specific waist circumference criteria $\geq$ 94 cm in Europoid men, $\geq$ 80 cm in Europoid women).

Plus two of the following:
1. Elevated triglycerides $\geq$ 1.7 mmol/L ($\geq$ 150 mg/dl) or on treatment for lipid abnormality.
2. Low HDL cholesterol < 1.03 mmol/L (40 mg/dl) in men, < 1.29 mmol/L (50 mg/dl) in women or on treatment for lipid abnormality.
3. Hypertension. Systolic > 130 mmHg and/or diastolic >85 mmHg or diagnosed hypertension.
4. Impaired fasting glycaemia. Fasting plasma glucose $\geq$ 5.6 mm/L (100 mg/dl) or diagnosed type 2 diabetes.

Family history of heart disease

Cardiovascular risk increases 1.5–1.7 fold with an affected first-degree male relative aged < 55 years or female relative aged < 65 years.

Homocysteine

Increased plasma concentrations of this sulphur-containing amino acid are associated with increased cardiovascular risk.
Normal plasma homocysteine concentration = 8–15 μmol/L

Moderate hyperhomocysteinaemia = 16–30 μmol/L
Intermediate hyperhomocysteinaemia = 31–100 μmol/L
Severe hyperhomocysteinaemia = >100 μmol/L

A 5 μmol/L rise in plasma homocysteine can increase cardiovascular risk by 20–30%.

Renal impairment

Cardiovascular risk increases 20–30-fold with the diagnosis of end-stage renal failure.

High-sensitivity C-reactive protein (hsCRP)

The acute phase, C-reactive protein can function as a marker for generalized inflammation which is a risk factor for cardiovascular disease. See Table 3.4.

Table 3.4 **High-sensitivity C-reactive protein (hsCRP) and risk**

hsCRP level	Risk
< 1.0 mg/L	Low
1.0–2.9 mg/dl	Intermediate
>3.0 mg/L	High

Cumulative risk scores

These integrate sex, age, smoking history, blood pressure and cholesterol profile to produce an estimated individual absolute 10-year risk of a cardiovascular event (myocardial infarction, stroke, angina and associated cardiovascular mortality) (Figure 3.1).

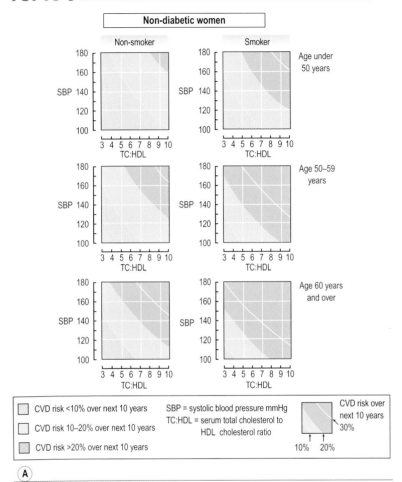

Figure 3.1 Cardiovascular risk prediction charts for non-diabetic women (A) and non-diabetic men (B).
Continued

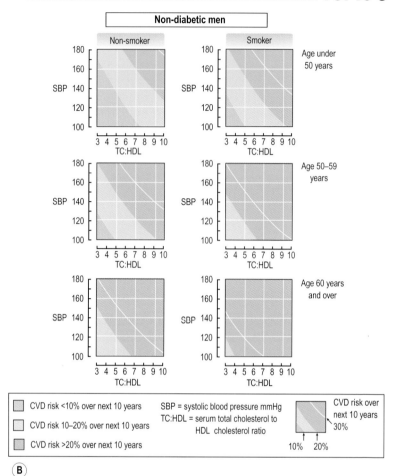

Figure 3.1—cont'd

TOPIC ❹

Electrophysiology

Topic Contents

Normal 12-lead ECG

Lead position

See Figure 4.1.

Cardiac axis

See Figure 4.2.
Normal axis: $-30°$ to $+90°$
Leftward axis: $-30°$ to $-90°$
Rightward axis: $+90°$ to $+180°$

Normal resting values

Adult resting heart rate: 50–100 beats per minute
ECG R-R interval (25 mm/s paper speed): each large square is 0.2 s; each small square is 0.04 s.
P wave (best seen lead II)
- Amplitude <2.5 mm.
- Duration <12 ms.
- Frontal plane axis 0 to $+75°$.
PR interval: 120–220 ms

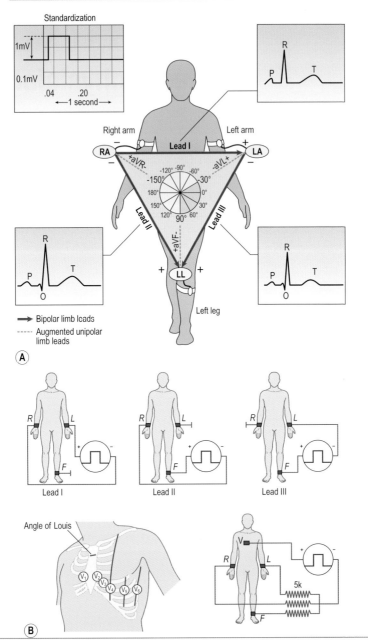

Figure 4.1 Standard ECG lead position. (A) Standard limb lead position with corresponding electrocardiographic vectors. (B) Standard praecordial chest lead position.

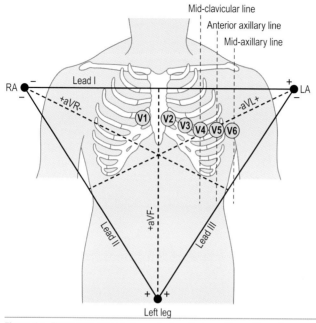

Figure 4.2 Einthoven's triangle demonstrating electrocardiographic vectors.

QRS
- Duration : <110 ms.
- Normal q wave duration < 0.04 s, amplitude < 25% of R wave.
- R waves begin in V1 or V2 and progress in size to V5 (R-V6 usually smaller than R-V5).
- S waves begin in V6 or V5 and progress in size to V2 (S-V1 usually smaller than S-V2).
- Usual transition from S>R in the right precordial leads to R>S in the left precordial leads is V3 or V4.

QT interval:
- Male: < 440 ms
- Female: < 460 ms
- QT interval corrected for heart rate (QTc) = QT/√RR

U wave
- Amplitude < 1/3 T wave amplitude in the same lead.
- Direction same as T wave direction in the same lead.
- Measurement of QT should not include U wave.
- U waves >1/3 T wave amplitude or merged into descending slope of T wave may be pathological.

Abnormalities of the 12-lead ECG

Atrial hypertrophy

Left:
- P wave in lead II > 2.5 mm
- and/or bifid and biphasic P wave in V1.

Right:
- P wave in leads II and V1 > 2.5 mm.
- QRS voltage in V1 < 5 mm and V2/V1 voltage ratio > 6.

Left ventricular hypertrophy (LVH)
- ESTES criteria for LVH ('diagnostic', >5 points; 'probable', 4 points).
- CORNELL voltage criteria for LVH (sensitivity = 22%, specificity = 95%).
  S in V3 + R in aVL > 28 mm (men) S in V3 + R in aVL > 20 mm (women).
- Other voltage criteria
  R wave in left precordial lead > 27 mm
  S wave in right precordial lead > 30 mm
  Sum of greatest R and S > 40 mm.

Right ventricular hypertrophy
Dominant R wave in V1 with normal QRS duration
Axis > +90°
ST segment depression V1–V3

Left bundle branch block
Usually abnormal
Prolonged QRS duration
Absence of q waves in leads I, aVL, V4–V6
Absence of secondary r (notch) wave in V1

Right bundle branch block
Normal finding in 10% of population
Prolonged QRS duration
Presence of secondary positive wave in V1

Stress ECG
Mortality rates <1/10 000 tests
Resting oxygen consumption = 3.5 ml/kg/min = 1 MET
Target heart rate = 85% maximum predicted heart
Maximum predicted heart rate = 220 − age (years) in males, 210 − age (years) females.

Bruce Protocol
See Table 2.1.

Pathological changes during exercise
ST segment depression
- Coronary disease likely if down-sloping ST segment depression >1.0 mm 80 ms after the J point.
- Ventricular arrhythmias (>10 premature ventricular beats per minute).
- Failure to increase systolic blood pressure with exercise.

Signal averaged ECG
This technique is used to detect low-amplitude surface electrograms which are undetectable by standard electrocardiography. These signals are associated with areas of slow conduction that occur following a myocardial infarction or in arrhythmogenic right ventricular cardiomyopathy (ARVC). Orthogonal XYZ leads are used to record signals which are averaged and filtered ($X^2 + Y^2 + Z^2$) to produce a root mean square voltage (RMS). A normal QRS duration is ≤ 114 ms and normal RMS amplitude in the terminal 40 ms is ≥ 20 μV.

In post-infarction patients, negative predictive value is >95% although positive predictive value is approximately 20% (Figure 4.3).

Signal Averaged ECG

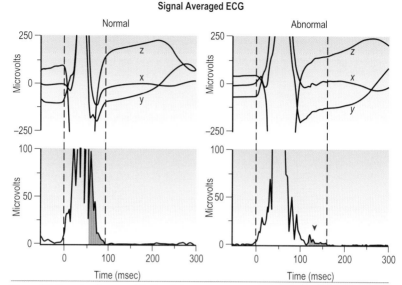

Figure 4.3 Example of a normal (left) and abnormal (right) signal averaged ECG.

T wave alternans

T wave alternans on the surface ECG is a beat-to-beat fluctuation in the shape or amplitude of the T wave, and reflects abnormal cardiomyocyte repolarization. A growing body of evidence suggests that it represents a risk marker for sudden cardiac death from ventricular tachyarrhythmias, particularly in patients with heart failure. T wave alternans develops at higher heart rates, particularly in a vulnerable zone above 95 bpm.

T wave alternans is measured using spectral analysis of the ECG and T wave.

A T wave alternans study provides either a **positive**, **negative** or **intermediate** result.

Positive
Sustained alternans with onset at HR <110 bpm.

Sustained alternans is defined as:
1. T wave alternans induced above of specific heart rate for a patient where HR <110 bpm.
2. At least one minute of electrical T wave alternans of >1.9 μV and alternans ratio >3.
3. Artefact-free data: <10% beats are ectopy, respiratory activity <0.25 cycles/beat, HR variation <30 bpm over 130 beats.

Negative
1. Does not meet the criteria of a positive test, and
2. Maximum HR achieved >105 bpm (see Figure 4.4).

Intermediate
1. Alternans free but maximum HR <105.
2. Alternans induced at HR >110.
3. ECG artefact, e.g. excessive ectopy, obscuring analysis.

T Wave Alternans

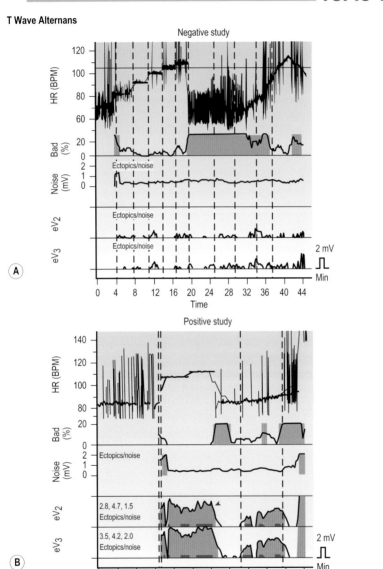

Figure 4.4 Example of normal/negative T wave alternans study (A) and abnormal/positive T wave alternans study (B).

Intracardiac electrograms

Normal conduction (Figure 4.5)

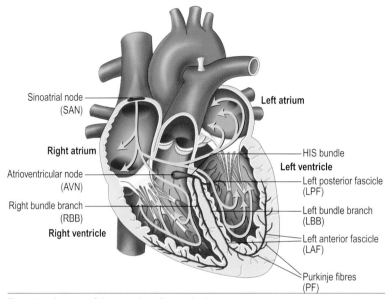

Figure 4.5 Anatomy of the normal cardiac conduction system.

Normal intracardiac intervals
PA: 25–55 ms
AH: 55–125 ms
HV: 35–55 ms
Sinus node recovery time (SNRT): < 150 ms
Sinoatrial conduction time (SACT): < 100 ms
AH 'jump': 50 ms increase in AH time for 10 ms decrease in pacing cycle.

Typical 4-wire EP study

High right atrium (HRA) – Quadrapolar catheter
Right ventricular apex (RVA) – Quadrapolar catheter
Coronary sinus (CS) – Decapolar catheter (wide-spaced)
His – Decapolar catheter (narrow-spaced).

Catheter position

See Figure 4.6.

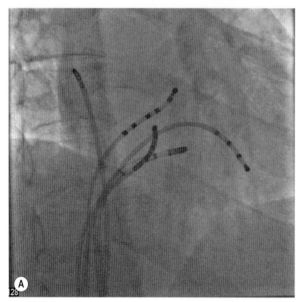

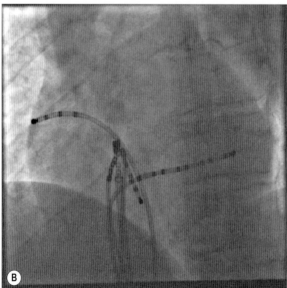

Figure 4.6 Catheter position for a 4-wire cardiac electrophysiological study. (A) RAO view. (B) LAO view.

Normal activation pattern

See Figure 4.7.

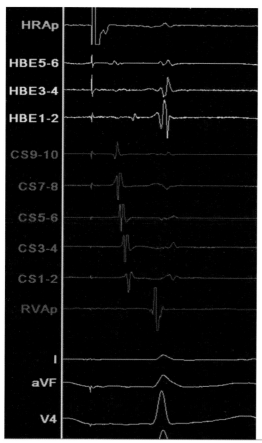

Figure 4.7 Intracardiac electrograms demonstrating the normal electrical activation pattern measured during a 4-wire electrophysiological study. Intracardiac electrogram nomenclature: HRA = high right atrium, HBE = His bundle electrogram, CS = coronary sinus, RVA = right ventricular apex. I, aVF and V4 are surface ECG leads.

Accessory pathways and Wolff-Parkinson-White syndrome

See Figures 4.8, 4.9, 4.10 for anatomical location of atrioventricular accessory pathways.

Pacemakers

See Table 4.1.

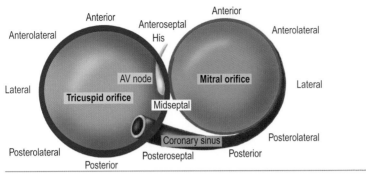

Figure 4.8 Schematic showing the anatomical location of atrioventricular accessory pathways in the plane of the atrioventricular valves.

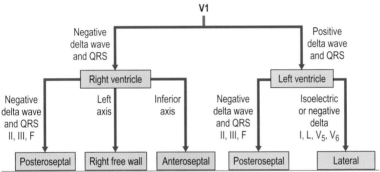

Figure 4.9 Guide for identification of accessory pathway location based upon 12-lead ECG abnormalities.

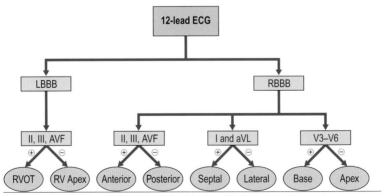

Figure 4.10 Identification of the anatomical origin of ventricular tachycardia based upon electrocardiographic appearance of the tachyarrhythmia on the 12-lead ECG.

Table 4.1 International pacemaker 4-letter code

Symbol	1st letter	2nd letter	3rd letter	4th letter	5th letter
Meaning	Paced chamber(s)	Sensed chamber(s)	Response to sensed beat (modes)	Additional programmable functions	Anti-tachycardia functions
Options	A = atrium V = ventricle D = dual 0 = none	A = atrium V = ventricle D = dual 0 = none	I = inhibited T = triggered D = dual 0 = none	R = rate response C = communicating M = multiprogrammable P = simple programmable 0 = none	P = paced S = shocks D = dual 0 = none

⑤ TOPIC

Ventricular function

Topic Contents

Chamber dimensions

M-mode echo (parasternal short axis):
Left ventricular internal diameters (LVIID):
End diastole (LVIDd): 3.5–5.6 cm
End systole (LVIDs): 1.9–4.0 cm
Left atrial diameter (end systole): 1.9–4.0 cm
Right ventricle: 0.7–2.3 cm
IVC: <1.5 cm

Table 5.1 Chamber volumes: Echocardiography and cardiac magnetic resonance

Left ventricle

Parameter (lower–upper 95% CI)	All		Male		Female	
	ECHO	CMR	ECHO	CMR	ECHO	CMR
EF (%)	>55	67 (58–76)	>55	67 (58–75)	>55	67 (58–76)
LVEDV (ml)	–	142 (102–183)	67–155	156 (115–198)	56–104	128 (88–168)
LVESV (ml)	–	47 (27–68)	22–58	53 (30–75)	19–49	42 (23–60)
SV (ml)	–	95	–	104	–	86
LV mass (g)	–	127 (90–164)	96–200	146 (108–184)	66–150	108 (72–144)

Right ventricle – CMR

Parameter (lower–upper 95% CI)	All	Male	Female
EF (%)	66 (54–78)	66 (53–78)	66 (54–68)
RVEDV (ml)	144 (98–190)	163 (113–213)	126 (84–168)
RVESV (ml)	50 (22–78)	57 (27–86)	43 (17–69)
RVSV (ml)	94 (64–124)	106 (72–140)	83 (57–108)
RV MASS (g)	48 (23–73)	66 (38–94)	48 (27–69)

Table 5.1 Continued

Right ventricle – Echo

	Right ventricle – Echo	
Basal RV diameter (cm)	Apical 4-chamber	2.0–2.8
Mid RV diameter (cm)		2.7–3.3
Apex–basal length (cm)		7.1–7.9
RVOT at AV level	Parasternal short axis	2.5–2.9
RVOT at PV annulus level		1.7–2.3
RV diastolic area (cm^2)		11–28
RV systolic area (cm^2)		7.5–6
RV fractional area change (%)		32–60
TAPSE*		16–20

Corrected for body surface area (BSA)

Parameter (lower–upper 95% CI)	All		Male		Female	
	ECHO	CMR	ECHO	CMR	ECHO	CMR
LVESV/BSA	12–30	26		27		24
LVEDV/BSA	35–75	78		80		75
LV MASS/BSA		69	50–102	74	44–88	63
RVESV/BSA		27 (13–41)		29 (14–43)		25 (12–38)
RVEDV/BSA		78 (57–99)		83 (60–106)		73 (55–92)
RV MASS/BSA		31		34		28

TAPSE = tricuspid annular plane systolic excursion.

Ventricular wall thickness and mass

Echo (parasternal long axis M-mode – see Figures 5.1 and 5.2)
Left ventricle (LV)
Posterior LV wall thickness (PWT) in systole (cm)
0.6–1.2; Hypertrophy $\geq$1.2

Interventricular septum (IVS) thickness in systole (cm)
0.6–1.2; Hypertrophy $\geq$1.2

LV mass (g) = 1.04 x [(IVS + LVEDD + PWT)^3 – LVEDD^3] – 13.6
LV mass index = LV mass corrected for BSA (g/m^2)
Mean (95%CI) = 87 (64–109)
Men > 102 g/m^2 = LVH
Women > 88 g/m^2 = LVH

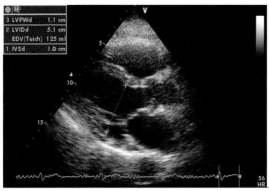

Figure 5.1 Parasternal long-axis echocardiogram demonstrating measurement of LV septal and posterior wall thickness and end diastolic diameter.

RV wall thickness in systole (cm)
0.2–0.5; Hypertrophy $\geq$0.5
RV mass index g/m^2
26 (17–34); Hypertrophy $\geq$35

Athlete's heart

It should be noted that highly trained athletes, particularly those competing in endurance sports, have cardiac measurements that fall outside the normal ranges quoted above. Studies suggest the majority of athletes' measurements fall within the following values, although a small proportion of athletes have greater values, and exclusion of underlying heart disease must be determined.
LA diameter: <4.5 cm
LVEDD: <6.0 cm
Posterior LV thickness: <1.3 cm

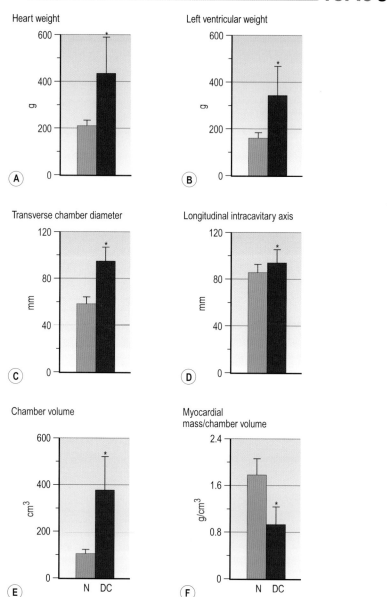

Figure 5.2 LV biometric data from normal (blue) and dilated cardiomyopathy (purple) hearts.

Cardiac cycle

Time intervals (see Figure 5.3)

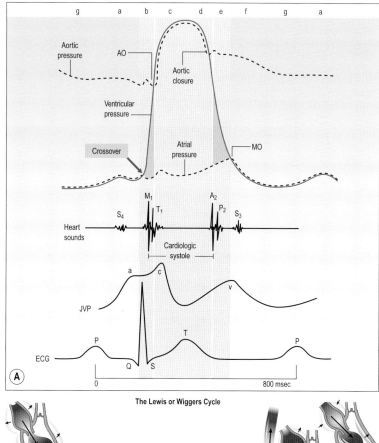

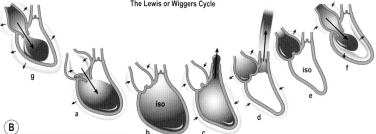

Figure 5.3 The normal cardiac cycle. (A) Schematic demonstrating the temporal relations of aortic pressure, left ventricular pressure, left atrial pressure, the phonocardiogram, the jugular venous pressure and the surface electrocardiogram during the cardiac cycle. (B) A schematic representation of left ventricular filling, ejection and isovolumic phases during the cardiac cycle.

The time intervals for the cardiac cycle are sensitive to heart rate. The following values are based upon a heart rate of 70 beats per minute:

Single complete cardiac cycle – duration $\sim$ 0.9 s with HR = 70 bpm
Diastole:

- Isovolumic relaxation 0.08 s
- Ventricular filling 0.5 s
  - Rapid passive filling 0.15 s
  - Slow passive filling 0.22 s
  - Atrial systole 0.13 s
- Isovolumic contraction 0.05 s

Systole:

- Ventricular ejection 0.3 s

Haemodynamics

Invasive measurements

Chamber	Systole	Diastole	Mean	SaO$_2$ (%)
Aorta	100–140	60–90	80–100	>95
LV	100–140	<12	–	>95
LA			6–12	>95
RV	15–25	0–7		75
RA			<7	75
PA	<25	<10	<15	75
PCW			<12	>95
SVC			6–12	75
IVC			6–12	65

Table 5.2 **Intracardiac pressures**

LV, left ventricle; LA, left atrium; RV, right ventricle; RA, right atrium; PA, pulmonary artery; PCW, pulmonary capillary wedge; SVC, superior vena cava; IVC, inferior vena cava.

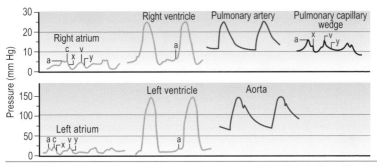

Figure 5.4 Schematic of the normal pressure tracings during cardiac catheterization of the right heart (above) and left heart (below).

Cardiac output calculations – Fick method

$$CO = O_2 \text{ consumption (ml/min)} / (AVO_2 \text{ difference (ml } O_2/100 \text{ ml blood}) \times 10$$
where normal O_2 consumption 3 ml O_2/kg or 125 ml/min/m^2

Arteriovenous oxygen difference (AVO$_2$ difference)
= arterial – mixed venous (PA) O_2 content, where O_2 content
= O_2 saturation × 1.34 × haemoglobin (g/dl)

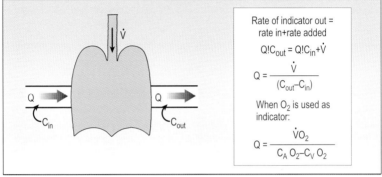

Figure 5.5 The Fick equation for calculation of cardiac output from arteriovenous oxygen gradient and VO$_2$.

Cardiac index (CI) in L/min/m^2 = CO/BSA – normal range $2.5-4.0$ L/min/m^2

Stroke volume index (SVI) = stroke volume/BSA – normal range $40-70$ ml

Stroke work index (SWI) in g/m/m^2 = mean LV systolic pressure
– mean LV diastolic pressure) × SVI × 0.0144

$$\text{Pulmonary arteriolar resistance (PAR)} = \frac{\text{mean PAP} - \text{ean LAP (or PCWP)}}{CO}$$

$$\text{Total pulmonary resistance (TPR)} = \frac{\text{mean PAP}}{CO}$$

$$\text{Systemic vascular resistance (SVR)} = \frac{\text{mean aortic BP} - \text{mean RAP}}{CO}$$

Table 5.3 **Normal ranges for cardiac output and resistance indices**	
Index	Normal range
Resting cardiac output (CO)	4–6 L/min
Cardiac index (CI)	2.5–4.0 L/min/m^2
Stroke volume (SV)	75–105 ml
Stroke volume index (SVI)	40–70 ml/m^2
Stroke work index (SWI)	40–80 g/m/m^2
Pulmonary vascular resistance (PVR)	<200 dynes/s/cm^{-5} <2.5 Wood units
Systemic vascular resistance (SVR)	770–1500 dynes/s/cm^{-5} 10–20 Wood units
Max LV dP/dt	1000–2400 mmHg/s

Pressure–volume analysis

Simultaneous pressure and volume recording using high-fidelity micromanometers and conductance catheters allows construction of pressure–volume loop relationships. These allow recording of PV relations during steady state and with dynamic manoeuvres such as preload or afterload alteration to provide load-independent measures of chamber function (see Figure 5.6).

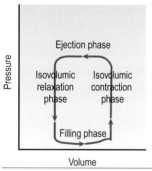
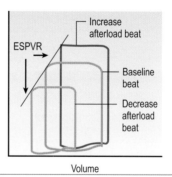

Figure 5.6 A schematic diagram of the normal left ventricular pressure–volume relationship during steady state recording of one cardiac cycle (left) and during variation in preload or afterload to calculate load-independent parameters, e.g. the end systolic pressure–volume relationship (ESPVR).

Table 5.4 **Normal values for pressure–volume analysis**			
LV	Diastole	Tau	40.8 ± 10.6 ms
		EDPVR – Po	−0.52 ± 5.9 mmHg
		EDPVR – β	0.036 ± 0.2 mmHg/ml
	Systole	ESPVR	2.1 ± 0.8 mmHg/ml
		PRSW	81.8 ± 10.4 mmHg
		dPdt max/EDV	18.7 ± 6.1 mmHg/s/ml
RV	Systole	RV elastance	1.3 ± 0.84 mmHg/ml

Non-invasive measurements

Echo

Fractional shortening (FS) is a common measure of left ventricular cavity changes during the cardiac cycle when measured using M-mode echo:

$$FS(\%) = \frac{LVEDD - LVESD}{LVEDD} \times 100$$

FS normal range $30-45\%$

Ejection fraction (EF) is the most common measurement used to report left ventricular function, and represents the % change in LV volume between systole and diastole. Simpson's rule is used to calculate LV volume and EF from 2D measurements. It derives volume from a cubic relationship, assuming the LV cavity is ellipsoidal (see Figure 5.7):

$$LVEDV = (LVEDD)^3$$

$$LVESV = (LVESD)^3$$

$$EF(\%) = \frac{(LVEDD)^3 - (LVESD)^3}{(LVEDD)^3} \times 100$$

EF $(\%)$ normal range $55-85\%$

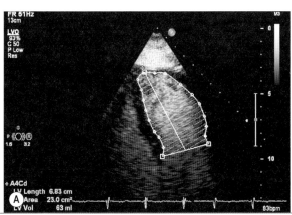

Figure 5.7 Contrast echocardiography to measure left ventricular volumes and ejection fraction using Simpson's rule from the apical 4-chamber view at end diastole (A) and end systole (B).

Continued

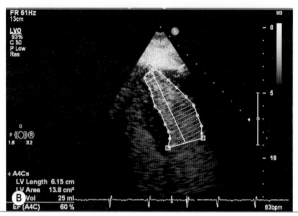

Figure 5.7—cont'd

Diastolic function

Doppler assessment of the transmitral filling pattern is a measure of ventricular diastolic compliance. The transmitral filling pattern consists of two waves, E and A (see Figures 5.8 and 5.9). The E wave reflects passive filling during early (auxotonic) diastole, and the A wave is generated by atrial systole ejecting blood into the ventricle.

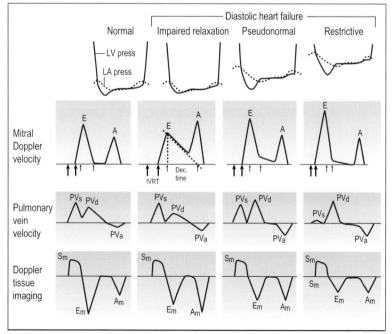

Figure 5.8 Schematic demonstrating normal and abnormal left ventricular diastolic physiology.

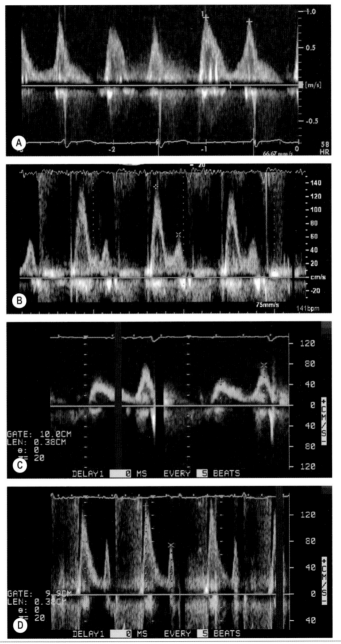

Figure 5.9 Doppler echocardiographic examples of transmitral left ventricular filling. A. Normal; B. Pseudonormal; C. E: A reversal; D. Restrictive.

The peak amplitude of the E and A waves, E wave deceleration time and the E:A ratio are measured to determine whether diastolic dysfunction is present. The E wave is usually greater than the A wave, but this varies with gender (see Table 5.5) and age (see Table 5.6). Peak E wave amplitude, E wave deceleration and the E:A ratio tend to fall with age in normal subject. This reflects the compliant younger ventricle, with 80–85% of diastolic filling occurring during the first two thirds of diastole. As the individual ages, atrial contraction contributes an increasing proportion of diastolic filling, with E and A waves peak velocities becoming equal (E:A ratio = 1) in the sixth or seventh decade.

Table 5.5 Normal transmitral Doppler flow indices and influence of gender

Parameter	Male	Female
Peak E wave (cm/s)	66 ± 15	70 ± 16
Peak A wave (cm/s)	67 ± 16	72 ± 18
E wave deceleration (s)	0.21 ± 0.04	0.19 ± 0.04
E:A ratio	1.04 ± 0.38	1.03 ± 0.34
E-at-A wave velocity (cm/s)	<20	<20

Table 5.6 Normal transmitral Doppler flow indices and influence of age

Parameter	Age (years) 2–20	21–40	41–60	>60
Peak E wave (cm/s)	88 ± 14	75 ± 13	71 ± 13	71 ± 11
Peak A wave (cm/s)	49 ± 12	51 ± 11	57 ± 13	75 ± 12
E wave deceleration (s)	0.14 ± 0.02	0.16 ± 0.01	0.18 ± 0.02	0.20 ± 0.3
E:A ratio	1.80	1.47	1.25	0.95
A wave duration (s)	0.113 ± 0.017	0.127 ± 0.013	0.133 ± 0.013	0.138 ± 0.019
IVRT (ms)	50 ± 9	67 ± 8	74 ± 7	87 ± 7

TOPIC 5

Left ventricular isovolumic relaxation time (IVRT)

Normal mean values in Table 5.6.
$<$60 ms – early MV opening – restrictive filling, or healthy young adults.
$>$100 ms – delayed relaxation and late MV opening.

PCWP estimation

$$\text{Mean PCWP} = 17 + (5 \times E/A) - (0.11 \times IVRT)(r = 0.88)$$

Tei Index

$$\text{Tei Index} = \frac{(IVCT + IVRT)}{ET}$$

$$IVCT = \text{Isovolumic ventricular contraction time}$$
$$IVRT = \text{Isovolumic ventricular relaxation time}$$
$$ET = \text{Ejection time}$$
$$\text{Normal LV Tei Index} = 0.38 \text{ abnormal} > 0.6$$
$$\text{Normal RV Tei Index} = 0.28$$

Colour M-mode Doppler

$$E = \text{peak Doppler E velocity}$$
$$Vp = \text{flow propagation velocity of early transmitral flow}$$
$$E/Vp \text{ ratio} - \text{normal} < 1.5$$
$$PCWP = 5.27 \times [E/Vp] + 4.6$$

Tissue Doppler

A normal spectral display recorded from the basal lateral left ventricular segment is presented in Figure 5.8.

$E'(E_M) = $ Peak velocity during early diastole (passive LV filling) – normal < 8 cm/s
$A_M = $ Peak velocity with atrial systole – normal
$S_M = $ Peak velocity with ventricular systole

E/E' ratio is a measurement used to predict LA pressure. Normal range <10.

Table 5.7 **Normal and abnormal tissue Doppler values evaluating left ventricular diastole**

Measurement		Normal	Mild diastolic dysfunction	Moderate diastolic dysfunction 'pseudonormalization'	Severe diastolic dysfunction	
					Reversible	Fixed/ restrictive
Mitral inflow	E/A	0.75<E/A<1.5	E/A<0.75	0.75< E/A<1.5	E/A>1.5	E/A>1.5
	DT(ms)	>140	>140	>140	<140	<140
Mitral inflow during Valsalva	ΔE/A from resting	<0.5	<0.5	>0.5	>0.5	<0.5
Tissue Doppler mitral annular motion	E/E' ratio	<10	<10	>10	>10	>10
Pulmonary venous flow	Systolic: diastolic ratio	S>D	S>D	S<D	S<D	S<D

Left atrial parameters

Table 5.8 **Normal values for left atrial size using M-mode echocardiography**

	Mean	Range (cm)
		Parasternal long axis
A-P diameter (cm)	3.0	2.3–3.8
S-I diameter (cm)	4.8	3.1–6.8
		Parasternal short axis
A-P diameter (cm)	2.9	2.2–4.1
M-L diameter (cm)	4.2	3.1–6.0
		Apical 4-chamber
S-I diameter (cm)	4.1	2.9–5.3
M-L diameter (cm)	3.8	2.9–4.9

	Normal	Mild-mod	Severe
LA area (cm^2)	<20	20–40	>40
LA volume	<60	60–78	>78
LA volume/BSA (ml/m^2)	<29	29–40	>40

Right atrial and right ventricular function

IVC collapse normally >50% with inspiratory effort if RA pressure <10 mmHg

Table 5.9 **Right atrial pressure estimation using IVC collapse and hepatic vein flow**

Mean RAP (mmHg)	IVC collapse (%)	Hepatic vein flow
0–5	>50	$V_S > V_D$
5–10	>50	$V_S = V_D$
10–15	<50	$V_S < V_D$
>20	<50	Diastolic flow only

In vivo haemodynamic monitoring

Table 5.10 **Intracardiac haemodynamic monitoring in patients with normal cardiac function**		
	24 hour ambulatory value (median)	Resting value (minimum nighttime)
RVSP (mmHg)	25	15
RVDP (mmHg)	4	1
ePAD (mmHg)	9	4
+RV dPdt (mmHg/s)	350	200

RVSP = right ventricular systolic pressure, RVDP = right ventricular diastolic pressure, estimated pulmonary artery diastolic pressure (ePAD) = RV pressure at point of PV opening = RV pressure at time of maximum +dPdt, +RV dPdt = maximum right ventricular dPdt.

Intrathoracic impedance monitoring

Normal threshold $<60\ \Omega\cdot d$ (76.9% sensitivity, 1.5 false positive results per patient year)

Radionuclide parameters of normal diastolic function

1. Peak filling rate (PFR) >2.5x EDV/s
2. Time to peak filling rate (TPFR) <180 ms
3. Filling fraction (%) at one third, one half and two thirds diastole
4. E:A ratio 1:40

MVO_2 exercise testing

Exercise testing can be used to measure maximal/peak oxygen uptake (MVO_2) (ml/kg/min), which may be limited by cardiac output, peripheral perfusion, impaired skeletal muscle metabolism, impaired respiratory function, test compliance or other issues. If the individual achieves maximal aerobic capacity during exercise, and utilizes anaerobic metabolism for further ATP generation, then they have reached their anaerobic threshold. At the anaerobic threshold CO_2 generation exceeds O_2 utilization, and the respiratory quotient (CO_2 produced/O_2 uptake = RQ) >1.0.

Normal MVO_2 range is dependent upon age, sex, height and weight, with values below 25 ml/kg/min suggestive of possible cardiac impairment. Given the variability of normal range, reporting absolute MVO_2 has limitations, although in patients with severe heart failure, a peak MVO_2 of <14 ml/kg/min is an independent predictor of poor survival and a criteria for referral for cardiac transplantation.

Reporting MVO_2 as a percentage of predicted MVO_2 for the individual is more useful:
- ≥80% predicted MVO_2 = normal test
- <80% predicted MVO_2 = abnormal test

If MVO_2 <80% predicted and RQ >1.05 – cardiac limitation of exercise.

If MVO_2 <80% predicted and RQ <1.05 – non cardiac limitation of exercise e.g. check FEV1/FVC.

Ventilatory efficiency is also impaired in heart failure. This is calculated from the slope of minute ventilation (V_E) vs CO_2 production (VCO_2).

$$V_E/VCO_2 \text{ slope} < 34 \text{ normal}$$

Serum natriuretic peptides

Two natriuretic peptides are available, brain natriuretic peptide (BNP) and N-terminal pro-brain natriuretic peptide (proNT-BNP).

Table 5.11 shows approximate normal and abnormal ranges for diagnosis of chronic heart failure in untreated patients, although these are sensitive to the assay and local laboratory values may vary. The sensitivity and specificity may also vary depending upon the value selected as upper limit of normal. The variation of sensitivity, specificity, positive predictive value (PPV), negative predictive value (NPV) and extrapolated accuracy for BNP in the diagnosis of chronic heart failure are also presented in Table 5.11 (see also Table 5.12).

Table 5.11 Normal ranges for serum natriuretic peptides

BNP			NT-proBNP		
Chronic HF unlikely	Intermediate range	Chronic HF likely	Chronic HF unlikely	Intermediate range	Chronic HF likely
<100 pg/ml	100–400 pg/ml	>400 pg/ml	<400 pg/ml	400–2000 pg/ml	>2000 pg/ml

Table 5.12 Diagnostic accuracy of various threshold values for serum brain natriuretic peptide to diagnose heart failure

Threshold (upper limit) pg/ml	Sensitivity	Specificity	PPV	NPV	Accuracy
50	97%	62%	71%	96%	79%
80	93%	74%	77%	92%	83%
100	90%	76%	79%	89%	83%
125	87%	79%	80%	87%	83%
150	85%	83%	83%	85%	84%

Dilated cardiomyopathy

The formal diagnosis requires the left ventricle to be dilated with the internal end-diastolic dimension (LVEDD) > 2.7 m^2 of body surface area and either ejection fraction < 45% or M-mode fractional shortening <30%. However, the normal distribution of ventricular dimension across the healthy population results in 1–2.5% of healthy individuals fitting either of these parameters (Figure 5.10).

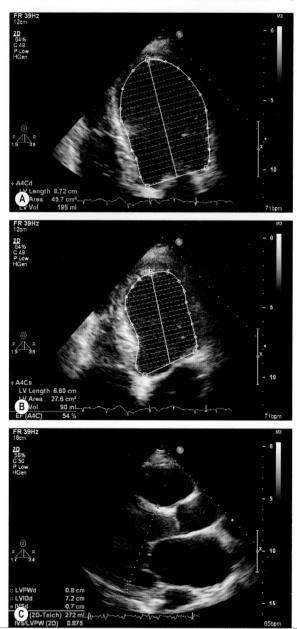

Figure 5.10 Apical 4-chamber view of a dilated left ventricle with end diastolic (A) and end systolic (B) volumes calculated using planimetry and Simpson's rule. (C) Parasternal short axis of a heart with dilated cardiomyopathy at end diastole.

Cardiac valvular structure and function

Topic Contents

Unidirectional flow of blood through the cardiac chambers is ensured by the presence of four cardiac valves which prevent backflow. Normal structure and function of the aortic, mitral, pulmonary and tricuspid valves is described, followed by normal values for the common prosthetic valves.

Table 6.1 **Normal values for mean and peak gradients and valve area for the four heart valves**

Valve	Aortic	Mitral	Pulmonary	Tricuspid
Peak jet velocity (m/s)	<1.3	0.9	<0.75	0.5
Peak gradient (mmHg)	<10	<3	<10	<3
Mean gradient (mmHg)	<10		<10	<1
Valve area (cm^2)	>2.0	4.0–6.0	>3.0	5.0–8.0

Aortic valve disease

$$\text{Peak gradient} = 4 \times \text{peak jet velocity}^2$$

$$\text{Aortic valve area} = \frac{\text{aortic valve flow(ml/s)}}{44.5 \times \sqrt{\text{mean aortic gradient}}}$$

Aortic stenosis

It is important to remember that these peak gradients/velocities depend upon preserved left ventricular systolic function. In the setting of impaired left ventricular function, acceleration of ejected blood from the LVOT (subvalvular) to AV by greater than four times (the dimensionless

Table 6.2 **Echocardiographic parameters for grading the severity of aortic stenosis**			
	Mild AS	Moderate AS	Severe AS
Peak jet velocity (m/s)	1.7–2.9	3.0–4.0	>4.0
Peak gradient (mmHg)	<36	36–64	≥64
Mean gradient (mmHg)	<25	25–40	>40
Valve area (cm^2)	1.5–2.0	1.0–1.5	<1.0

index) is suggestive of significant aortic stenosis, and dobutamine stress echocardiography is indicated.

$$\text{Dimensionless index (velocity ratio)} = \text{peak LVOT velocity/peak AV velocity}$$
$$\text{Normal} = 1{:}1 \ (1)$$
$$\text{Severe AS} = {<}1{:}4 \ ({<}0.25)$$

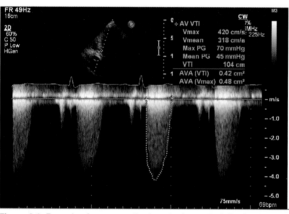

Figure 6.1 Example of severe aortic stenosis demonstrated using transaortic continuous wave Doppler

Aortic regurgitation

Table 6.3 Echocardiographic parameters for grading severity of aortic valve regurgitation

	Mild AR	Moderate AR	Severe AR
Angiographic grade	1	2	3+
Colour Doppler jet width (% LVOT diameter)	Central jet <25%	25–65	>65
Doppler vena contracta width (cm)	<0.3	0.3–0.6	>0.6
Regurgitant fraction (%)	<30	30–49	>50
AR deceleration rate (m/s^2)	<2	2–3	>3
Pressure half time (ms)	>500	250–500	<250
Regurgitant orifice area (cm^2)	<0.1	0.1–0.29	>0.3
VTI diastolic flow reversal in descending aorta (cm)			>15

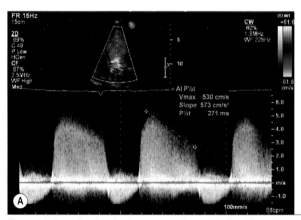

Figure 6.2 Example of moderate–severe aortic regurgitation. (A) Continuous wave Doppler tracing demonstrating pressure half time.

Continued

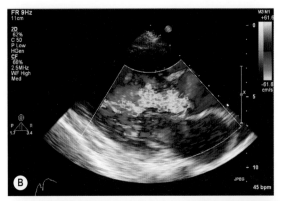

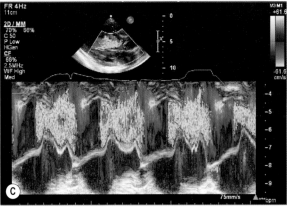

Figure 6.2—cont'd (B) Colour Doppler and (C) colour M-mode demonstrating the size of the regurgitant jet relative to the aortic valve orifice and left ventricular outflow tract.

Mitral stenosis

Table 6.4 **Echocardiographic parameters for grading severity of mitral valve stenosis**

	Mild MS	Moderate MS	Severe MS
Valve area (cm²)	1.6–2.0	1.0–1.5	<1.0
Mean pressure gradient (mmHg)	<5	5–10	>10
Pressure half time (ms)	70–139	140–219	>220
PAP (mmHg)	<30	30–49	>50

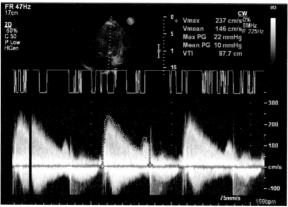

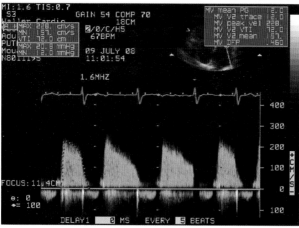

Figure 6.3 Pulse wave Doppler images demonstrating transmitral diastolic flow in patients with severe mitral stenosis. (A) Example in sinus rhythm. (B) Example in atrial fibrillation, when the mean pressure gradient from several cardiac cycles is required.

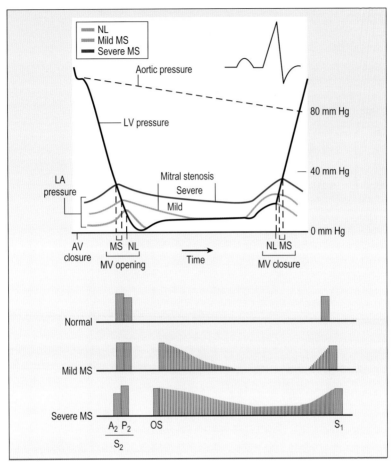

Figure 6.4 Schematic demonstrating (A) left atrial and left ventricular pressure tracings during normal, mild, moderate and severe mitral stenosis; and (B) heart sounds and murmurs heard on auscultation of the normal heart, and hearts with mild and severe mitral stenosis.

Mitral regurgitation

Table 6.5 **Echocardiographic parameters for grading severity of mitral valve regurgitation**

	Mild MR	Moderate MR	Severe MR
Angiographic grade	1	2	3+
Colour Doppler jet area (cm^2)	<4	4–10	>10
Colour Doppler jet area (%LA)	<20%	20–40%	>40%
Doppler vena contracta width (cm)	<0.3	0.3–0.69	≥0.70
PISA radius (Nyquist 40 cm/s)	<0.4	0.41–0.99	>1.0
Regurgitant volume (ml/beat)	<30	30–59	≥60
Regurgitant fraction (%)	<30	30–49	≥50
Regurgitant orifice area (cm^2)	<0.2	0.2–0.4	>0.4

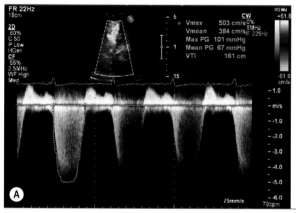

Figure 6.5 Severe mitral regurgitation. (A) Continuous wave Doppler tracing of MR jet with measurement of the velocity time integral (VTI).

Continued

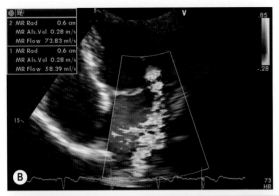

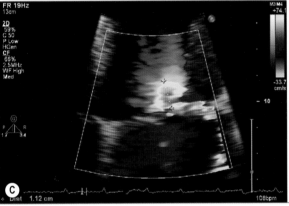

Figure 6.5—cont'd (B, C) Examples of PISA measurement using colour Doppler at the mitral valve regurgitant orifice.

Pulmonary stenosis

PS is diagnosed when peak jet velocity is >3 m/s, corresponding to a peak PV gradient of 36 mmHg.

Moderate PS peak gradient 40–74 mmHg

Severe PS peak gradient >75 mmHg

Pulmonary regurgitation

Treatment of PR is currently based on symptoms rather than severity scales, although other factors including RV function and QRSD are important variables in timing replacement.

Table 6.6 **Echocardiographic parameters for grading severity of pulmonary valve regurgitation**

	Mild	Moderate	Severe
Jet size (cm)	<1.0	Intermediate	Wide
Regurgitant fraction (%)	<40	40–59	>60
CW jet density/deceleration rate	Soft/slow	Dense/variable	Dense/steep
$RVOT_{VTI}/LVOT_{VTI}$	= or +	++	+++

Tricuspid stenosis

Normal TV area is $\sim$7.0 cm^2.
Severe tricuspid stenosis is rare, and is diagnosed when the TV area is less than 1 cm^2, resulting in a pressure drop of >5 mmHg.

Tricuspid regurgitation

Tricuspid regurgitation is relatively common, reflecting tricuspid annular dilatation secondary to right ventricular dilatation as a result of pulmonary hypertension.

The peak velocity of the TR jet can be used as an indirect measure of PA pressure, as it reflects the pressure difference between the RV and RA.

RV pressure = PA pressure during RV systole
$$PA\ pressure = (4 \times peak\ TR\ velocity^2) + RA\ pressure\ (CVP)$$

Table 6.7 **Echocardiographic parameters for grading severity of tricuspid valve regurgitation**

	Mild	Moderate	Severe
Jet area (cm^2)	<5	5.1–9.9	>10
Vena contracta width (cm)		<0.7	>0.7
PISA radius (cm)	<0.5	0.5–0.9	>0.9
CW jet density/contour	Soft/parabolic	Dense/variable	Dense/triangular
RA/RV/IVC size	Normal	Normal/dilated	Dilated
Hepatic vein flow	Systolic dominance	Systolic blunted	Systolic reversal

Prosthetic heart valves

Subtypes:
Mechanical – caged ball, monoleaflet, bileaflet
Biological – stented, stentless, percutaneous

Size chosen to provide the largest effective orifice area (EOA) in relation to the patient's valve annulus size.

Normal reference values of EOAs are presented in Table 6.8 for aortic valve prostheses, and in Table 6.9 for mitral valve prostheses. Threshold for prosthetic valve – patient mismatched sizing are presented in Table 6.10.

Table 6.8 **Effective orifice area values for the different sizes of commonly used aortic valve prostheses**

	Prosthetic valve size (mm)					
	19	21	23	25	27	29
Aortic mechanical prostheses						
St. Jude Medical Standard	1.0	1.4	1.5	2.1	2.7	3.2
St. Jude Medical Regent	1.6	2.0	2.2	2.5	3.6	4.4
Carbomedics Standard	1.0	1.5	1.7	2.0	2.5	2.6
Medtronic Advantage	-	1.7	2.2	2.8	3.3	3.9
Aortic stented bioprostheses						
Mosaic	1.1	1.2	1.4	1.7	1.8	2.0
Carpentier-Edwards Perimount	1.1	1.3	1.5	1.8	2.1	2.2
Hancock II	-	1.2	1.3	1.5	1.6	1.6
Aortic stentless bioprostheses						
Medtronic Freestyle	1.2	1.4	1.5	2.0	2.3	
St. Jude Medical Toronto SPV	-	1.3	1.5	1.7	2.1	2.7

Table 6.9 Effective orifice area values for the different sizes of commonly used mitral valve prostheses

	Prosthetic valve size (mm)				
	25	27	29	31	33
Mitral mechanical prostheses					
St. Jude Medical Standard	1.5	1.7	1.8	2.0	2.0
MCRI On-X	2.2	2.2	2.2	2.2	2.2
Mitral stented bioprostheses					
Carpentier-Edwards Perimount	1.6	1.8	2.1	–	–
Hancock II	1.5	1.8	1.9	2.6	2.6
Medtronic Mosaic	1.5	1.7	1.9	1.9	–

Table 6.10 Threshold values of body surface area-indexed prosthetic valve EOA for diagnosis of prosthesis–patient mismatch (PPM)

	Normal/ mild (cm^2/m^2)	Moderate (cm^2/m^2)	Severe (cm^2/m^2)
Aortic prosthesis	>0.85	0.65–0.85	<0.65
Mitral prosthesis	>1.2	0.9–1.2	<0.9

Percutaneous aortic valve bioprostheses

Edwards-Sapien – 23 mm and 26 mm

CoreValve bioprostheses exists in two sizes according to the ascending aortic diameter (<35 mm or <45 mm) and one size for the aortic annulus (23 mm).

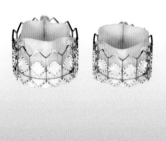

Figure 6.6 Edwards-Sapien Transcatheter Percutaneous Aortic Valves: 26 mm (left) and 23 mm (right). Courtesy of Edwards-Sapien.

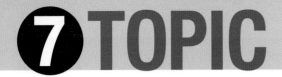

TOPIC 7

Pericardial structure and function

The normal pericardium is ~2 mm thick, and consists of three layers: the outer fibrous pericardium, and the inner serous pericardium, which is divided into visceral and parietal layers. The visceral serous pericardium forms the epicardial surface, and the parietal serous pericardium lines the fibrous pericardium.

The visceral serous pericardium covers the left and right ventricles, and right atrium. It extends over the first 1–2 cm of the great vessels entering and leaving the heart, before reflecting back as the parietal serous pericardium. Posterior to the left atrium, the reflection occurs at the oblique sinus, leaving the posterior aspect of the left atrium as extrapericardial (see Figure 7.1).

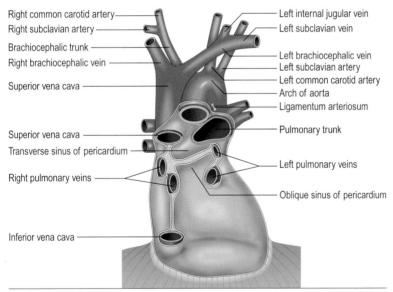

Right common carotid artery —
Right subclavian artery —
Brachiocephalic trunk —
Right brachiocephalic vein —
Superior vena cava —
Superior vena cava —
Transverse sinus of pericardium —
Right pulmonary veins —
Inferior vena cava —

— Left internal jugular vein
— Left subclavian vein
— Left brachiocephalic vein
— Left subclavian artery
— Left common carotid artery
— Arch of aorta
— Ligamentum arteriosum
— Pulmonary trunk
— Left pulmonary veins
— Oblique sinus of pericardium

Figure 7.1 Schematic of the pericardial anatomy and reflections on the posterior aspect of the normal heart.

The pericardial space normally contains <50 ml of serous fluid. An increase in pericardial fluid volume is known as a pericardial effusion.

The pericardium is normally compliant and flexible, transmitting intrathoracic pressure changes to the cardiac chambers within. The normal parietal pericardium has a tensile strength similar to rubber. Small distending forces lead to large amounts of stretch. As the pericardium stretches, stiffening increases, and it progressively resists further distension.

Therefore the pericardium restricts acute ventricular dilatation. In contrast, slowly accumulating effusions can stretch the pericardial sac, allowing potentially large volumes of fluid (>1.5 L) to be contained without significant intrapericardial pressure rises. However, once a stretch limit is reached, chronic accumulating fluid will rapidly increase pericardial pressure (from <5 mmHg up to 20 mmHg), with the development of cardiac tamponade.

Thickening and rigidity of the pericardial sac following chronic inflammation, for example from post pericardiotomy or tuberculous pericarditis, may result in loss of normal compliance.

The outcome is constrictive pericarditis (CP), which is characterized by two pathophysiological phenomena:
• Dissociation between the intrathoracic and intracardiac pressures.
• Interventricular dependence.

The characteristic physiological finding is a failure of the normal pressure gradient driving PV–LA–LV blood flow and left ventricular filling during inspiration. This leads to equalization of LV, LA/PCWP and RV diastolic pressures, with impairment of LV filling during inspiration. This is further exacerbated by increased RV filling, with bowing of the interventricular septum to the left.

Conversely during expiration LV filling increases, the septum is shifted to the right impairing RV filling within the fixed volume of the rigid pericardial sac. The movement of the septum from left to right and back with the respiratory cycle is detectable using echocardiography or CMR as the characteristic septal 'bounce'.

The pericardium appears thicker (>2 mm), and may be calcified. Further suggestive features include IVC dilatation, reversal of hepatic or IVC venous flow during diastole. Normally diastolic forward flow is greater than systolic forward flow in the hepatic veins. In constrictive pericarditis (and restrictive cardiomyopathy) hepatic veins, IVC and SVC are dilated, without inspiratory collapse. Hepatic vein diastolic flow reversal may be detectable in addition to forward flow, particularly during inspiration, whereas flow reversal is absent in the normal heart. In the SVC this inspiratory flow reversal may be evident, and underlies the basis for Kussmaul's sign.

Differentiating CP from restrictive cardiomyopathy (RCM) is a classical clinical challenge, as both conditions have similar/overlapping physiology, signs and investigations. Tissue Doppler may be helpful, as mitral annular motion is generally increased in CP, whereas it is significantly reduced in myocardial disease states including RCM. The early diastolic velocity E' is increased in CP, and reduced below 7 cm/s (normal >7 cm/s) in myocardial disease. Therefore an increased E' >7 cm/s in the setting of a restrictive filling pattern (E/A > 1.5, E deceleration time <160 ms) is suggestive of CP rather than myocardial disease.

The E/E' ratio is increased in CP, and is inversely proportional to PCWP (annulus paradoxus).

8 TOPIC

Adult congenital heart disease

Topic Contents

Genetic and non-genetic associations with congenital heart disease

Genetic

Table 8.1 Genetic syndromes associated with congenital heart disease

Syndrome	Typical genetic defect	Typical cardiac defects
Down syndrome	Trisomy 21	Atrioventricular septal defect, VSD, ASD, PDA
Holt–Oram syndrome	12q2	ASD, VSD
Turner syndrome	XO	Aortic coarctation, bicuspid aortic valve
Noonan syndrome	12q	Pulmonary stenosis, hypertrophic cardiomyopathy
Di George syndrome	22q11 deletion	Truncus arteriosus, tetralogy of Fallot, interrupted aortic arch
Williams syndrome	7q11 deletion	Supravalvular aortic stenosis, peripheral pulmonary artery stenosis

Non-genetic

Table 8.2 Non-genetic associations with congenital heart disease (known or suspected maternal factors)

Infective	Rubella, toxoplasmosis, Coxsackie B virus
Environmental	Trichloroethylene, dichloroethylene, chromium
Iatrogenic	Antiepileptics, lithium, thalidomide, warfarin, isotretinoin
Lifestyle	Alcohol and illicit drug use, low folate intake
Medical	Diabetes mellitus, phenylketonuria

Atrial septal defect (ASD)

Communication between the atrial chambers allowing mixing of blood.

Types of ASD (Figure 8.1)

Ostium secundum
Ostium primum
Sinus venosus defect
Coronary sinus ASD.

Ostium secundum defect

May present in adulthood with first occurrence of symptoms.
Defect in the area of fossa ovalis. May be amenable to transcatheter closure.

Ostium primum defect

This is part of a spectrum of atrioventricular septal defects, resulting from defective fusion of the inferior and superior endocardial cushions, leading to a common atrioventricular junction. Associated atrioventricular valve, atrial septal and ventricular septal anomalies can occur within this spectrum.
Associated with Down syndrome.
Definitive management is surgical. Repaired patients may present later with left atrioventricular valve regurgitation or, less commonly, left ventricular outflow tract obstruction.

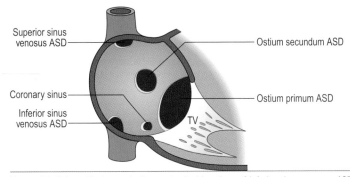

Figure 8.1 Schematic demonstrating anatomical locations of inferior sinus venosus ASD. TV, Tricuspid valve.

Sinus venosus defect

The defect lies in the majority of cases at the mouth of the superior vena cava (superior sinus venosus) and is frequently associated with anomalous drainage of the right upper pulmonary vein into the right atrium. Rarely the defect lies next to the inferior vena cava (inferior sinus venosus).

Definitive management is surgical.

Coronary sinus ASD

At least part of the wall between the coronary sinus and LA is absent. Often associated with a persistent left superior vena cava. Similar clinical course to secundum ASD, also dependent on size of defect and shunt.

Definitive management is surgical.

Clinical features

May be asymptomatic and discovered incidentally, but symptoms appear increasingly with age. Presentation includes:
Atrial fibrillation, atrial flutter, sick sinus syndrome
Right heart volume overload/right heart failure
Exertional dyspnoea
Recurrent chest infection
Paradoxical emboli
Pulmonary hypertension (ASD is associated with pulmonary hypertension though there is not thought to be a direct causal relationship)
Cyanosis.

Indications for closure

Right heart volume overload
ASD minimum diameter 10 mm
Left to right shunt > 1.5:1
Paradoxical emboli.

Before closure need to assess for: presence of significant pulmonary hypertension (precludes closure), presence of significant mitral valve disease (severity may be underestimated and may cause decompensation following closure).

The prognostic benefit of closure is reduced with increased age, though this does not preclude intervention. Delayed closure is associated with an increased risk of long term complications including atrial arrhythmias and reduced survival.

Ventricular septal defect (VSD)

Types of VSD

Membranous
Outlet
Inlet
Muscular.

Membranous (perimembranous/infracristal)

Most common.
Beneath crista supraventricularis, posterior to papillary muscle of conus, beneath aortic valve
Associated tricuspid valve abnormalities.

Outlet (supracristal/infundibular/doubly committed subarterial)

Located between crista supraventricularis and pulmonary valve. Right coronary cusp of aortic valve may prolapse into VSD leading to aortic regurgitation/subpulmonary stenosis.

Inlet

Defect in central fibrous body between tricuspid and mitral valves.
Often associated defects.

Muscular

Often multiple; in muscular septum.

Clinical features

Clinical features depend upon the anatomy and haemodynamic severity of the VSD and presence of associated anomalies.

VSDs can be classified according to haemodynamic effect. The measured variables are the pulmonary artery: aortic systolic pressure ratio and pulmonary blood flow: systemic blood flow ratio.

Small: Pressure ratio $<$ 0.3 and flow ratio $<$ 1.4
Moderate: Pressure ratio $>$ 0.3 and flow ratio 1.4 to 2.2
Large: Pressure ratio $>$ 0.3 and flow ratio $>$ 2.2
Eisenmenger: Pressure ratio $>$ 0.9 and flow ratio $<$ 1.5
Where the right ventricular systolic pressure is lower than left ventricular systolic pressure, in the absence of right ventricular outflow tract obstruction, the VSD is termed "restrictive"

Adults may have a small unrepaired VSD, a repaired VSD or Eisenmenger syndrome. Moderate or large VSDs are likely to have been repaired in childhood. Haemodynamically significant VSDs can lead to left heart pressure loading, right heart volume loading, pulmonary vascular disease and Eisenmenger syndrome.

Other complications include:
Infective endocarditis.
Aortic regurgitation due to aortic cusp prolapse (outlet VSD and membranous VSD).
Arrhythmia: Atrial fibrillation may occur with left atrial dilatation secondary to left heart volume overload. Ventricular arrhythmia and late sudden death are reported.
Right ventricular outflow obstruction. It may take the form of a 'double chamber right ventricle' in which muscular bands divide the right ventricle into a high-pressure proximal chamber and lower pressure distal chamber.

Indications for adult intervention include:

Significant left to right shunt (Qp/Qs $>$ 2)
Pulmonary artery systolic pressure $>$ 50 mmHg. If the pulmonary artery pressure (or arteriolar resistance) is greater than 2/3 systemic arterial pressure (or arteriolar resistance), there must be evidence of a net left to right shunt of $\geq$ 1.5 or evidence of reactivity or potential reversibility (assessment with pulmonary vasodilator or lung biopsy).
Ventricular dysfunction (left ventricular volume overload or right ventricular pressure overload)
Aortic cusp prolapse with greater than mild aortic incompetence
Significant right ventricular outflow tract obstruction (mean gradient $>$ 50 mmHg).

Patent ductus arteriosus (PDA)

The ductus arteriosus allows oxygenated blood to pass from the placenta to the aorta, bypassing the lungs in utero. The pulmonary end is situated just left of the bifurcation of the main pulmonary artery and connects to the descending aorta, distal to the left subclavian artery. It normally closes shortly after birth. Persistence of the ductus is associated with congenital rubella and is more common after premature birth. It may be present with other cardiac anomalies and in some cases is essential for survival.

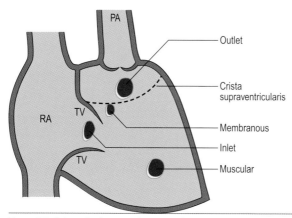

Figure 8.2 Schematic demonstrating anatomical locations of ventricular septal defects. RA = right atrium, TV = tricuspid valve leaflets, PA = pulmonary artery.

Clinical features

After birth the shunt direction reverses with changes in systemic and pulmonary pressures.

Large isolated PDAs are characterized by heart failure in infancy.

A PDA may be clinically silent throughout life or may not present till adulthood.

If the PDA is very small or operated early in childhood, normal survival can be expected.

Complications in unoperated or late operation of a significant PDA can include left atrial dilatation and atrial arrhythmia, left heart failure, pulmonary hypertension and Eisenmenger syndrome. If Eisenmenger syndrome occurs, deoxygenated blood via the PDA supplies lower extremities whilst the oxygenated aortic blood supplies the upper body (differential cyanosis).

Management

Selected adult cases for surgical or transcatheter closure.

Irreversible pulmonary hypertension should be excluded before closure of sizeable ducts. Closure is not always performed in clinically silent PDAs.

Coarctation of the aorta

A narrowing in the aorta, usually just distal to the left subclavian artery and at the level of the ductus arteriosus (or ligamentum arteriosum).

Associations include:

Bicuspid aortic valve, VSD, subvalvular aortic stenosis, mitral valve abnormalities
Circle of Willis aneurysm
Turner syndrome.

Clinical features

Presentation is dependent on the degree and site of obstruction, presence of associated congenital heart defects and collaterals which may mask the severity of the obstruction.

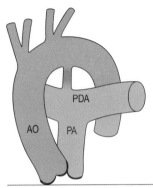

Figure 8.3 Patent ductus arteriosus: AO: Aorta; PA: Pulmonary artery.

Most adults with aortic coarctation have been previously operated. Untreated adults typically present with systemic arterial hypertension or less commonly with a murmur or symptoms such as headache or exertional leg discomfort. Occasionally angina or left ventricular failure will occur. Repair of the lesion should not be considered curative as late complications are common and include recoarctation, aneurysm formation (especially following Dacron patch aortoplasty), persistent systemic arterial hypertension (even in the absence of residual significant coarctation) and premature atherosclerosis with associated increased risk of cardiovascular events. Additional complications can arise from associated lesions.

Management

A pullback gradient of > 20 mmHg at catheterization is usually considered significant (in the absence of well-developed collaterals).

Percutaneous and surgical options are available for repair.

Surgical techniques include: resection with end-to-end anastomosis, subclavian flap aortoplasty (not recommended in adults), patch aortoplasty, interposition tube grafting and bypass (jump) grafting.

Usually infants and children undergo surgical repair.

Adults with previously unoperated native coarctation or with recoarctation may be suitable for transcatheter stenting.

Bicuspid aortic valve

1–2% of the population have a bicuspid aortic valve.

This is the most common cause of congenital aortic stenosis and results from commissural fusion of two valve leaflets. Associated anomalies include aortic coarctation, PDA and VSD. The natural history includes development of aortic stenosis or regurgitation (sometimes following infective endocarditis). There is also an associated abnormality of aortic root tissue, which increases risk of aortic aneurysm formation and aortic dissection.

Treatment options include: balloon valvuloplasty (children), open aortotomy (children), prosthetic valve replacement, Ross procedure.

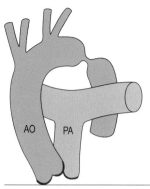

Figure 8.4 Schematic demonstrating anatomical location of coarctation of the aorta.

Subvalvular aortic stenosis

Typically a thin membrane or fibromuscular ridge in the left ventricular outflow tract. Occasionally takes the form of a fibromuscular tunnel or ring.

Associated lesions include VSD, bicuspid aortic valve and aortic coarctation.

Clinical features include secondary left ventricular hypertrophy and aortic regurgitation (due to damage from turbulent flow).

Subvalvular stenosis is often progressive and not uncommonly recurs after surgical repair.

Intervention may be considered if:
   symptomatic
   catheter or mean echo gradient > 50 mmHg (the gradient may be underestimated in the presence of a VSD).
   evidence of progressive, greater than mild aortic regurgitation.

Supravalvular aortic stenosis

Rare.
Associated with Williams syndrome.
It can take various forms and may be focal or diffuse. It is usually localized at the level of the sinotubular junction.
Other major vessels may be stenosed, including branch pulmonary arteries, carotid arteries and other systemic arterial vessels. The coronary arteries may be dilated and are also prone to accelerated atherosclerosis as they are exposed to high pressure proximal to the stenosis.

Intervention may be considered if the catheter or mean echo gradient > 50 mmHg.

Pulmonary stenosis

Pulmonary valve stenosis is the most common form of right ventricular outflow tract obstruction. It usually occurs in isolation and in most cases the valve is dome shaped with fused commissures.

Subvalvular pulmonary stenosis typically occurs in tetralogy of Fallot and in association with VSD. Double chambered right ventricle is a form of subinfundibular right ventricular outflow tract obstruction resulting from prominent right ventricular muscle bands.

Supravalvular pulmonary stenosis is associated with tetralogy of Fallot, Williams syndrome, Noonans syndrome and maternal rubella. It can also occur iatrogenically following pulmonary artery banding or arterial switch for transposition of the great arteries.

Haemodynamic severity is graded according to the peak systolic pressure gradient on cardiac catheterization. It provides an important guide for management decisions.

Trivial: < 25 mmHg

Mild: 25–49 mmHg

Moderate: 50–79 mmHg

Severe or Critical: > 80 mmHg

Indications for intervention include:
Pullback gradient at catheterization of > 50 mmHg
Symptomatic
Significant arrhythmia
Presence of right to left shunt (e.g. associated ASD)
Double chambered right ventricle with mid cavity gradient at catheterization > 50 mmHg

Pulmonary valve stenosis is often amenable to transcatheter balloon valvuloplasty. If pulmonary valve replacement is required, a human homograft is often used.

Ebstein anomaly

Describes apical displacement of the septal and posterior tricuspid valve leaflets with variable displacement and dysplasia of the anterior leaflet. There are varying degrees of tricuspid regurgitation.

Associated lesions include ASD, pulmonary stenosis and accessory conduction pathways. It is also seen in corrected transposition of the great arteries.

There is a spectrum of severity, which largely depends on the degree of leaflet displacement and tricuspid regurgitation and presence of associated lesions. In infancy it may present with heart failure and cyanosis with poor prognosis. Milder forms can be asymptomatic throughout life. Adults may develop exercise intolerance or symptomatic arrhythmia. Sudden death is also reported and thought to be arrhythmic. In the presence of an atrial septal defect there may be cyanosis or paradoxical embolic events.

In severe cases a bidirectional Glenn shunt or modified Fontan may be performed and the patient managed as for univentricular circulation. Less severe cases may be suitable for tricuspid valve replacement or repair.

Tetralogy of Fallot

The most common congenital cyanotic heart disease in adults.

The four components of the tetralogy are: infundibular right ventricular outflow tract obstruction $\pm$ valvular and supravalvular pulmonary stenosis, right ventricular hypertrophy, perimembranous VSD, aorta overriding interventricular septum (Figure 8.5).

There is a spectrum of severity. The majority of cases present early with cyanosis. With mild right ventricular outflow tract obstruction, the occasional patient will present in adulthood

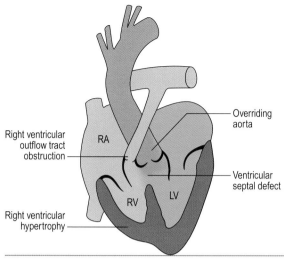

Figure 8.5 Schematic demonstrating the cardiac abnormalities associated with tetralogy of Fallot.

('pink tetralogy'). An extreme variant is pulmonary atresia with VSD in which the right ventricular outflow tract is atretic and pulmonary blood flow is obtained from major aortopulmonary collaterals (MAPCAs), patent ductus arteriosus or other acquired collaterals.

Today, most adults have been surgically repaired or, less commonly, shunt-palliated. Rarely, adults are previously unoperated.

Associated anomalies include:
Right side aortic arch
Coronary artery anomalies
ASD (pentalogy of Fallot)
Second VSD

Palliative procedures

Anastomosis of systemic to pulmonary circulation to increase pulmonary blood flow and include:

Blalock-Taussig shunt: subclavian artery to pulmonary artery (now modified)

Waterston anastomosis: right PA to ascending aorta (historical)

Potts anastomosis: left PA to descending aorta (historical)

Brock procedure: resection of right ventricular infundibular obstructive tissue (historical).

Corrective surgery

Now performed in infancy.

VSD closed.

Right ventricular outflow tract reconstruction: this may involve resection of infundibular obstructive tissue and patch placement to augment outflow. A transannular patch (crossing the pulmonary valve annulus) may need to be placed but is avoided where possible. In some cases, such as in pulmonary atresia, a right ventricular to pulmonary artery extracardiac conduit may be formed.

Outcome

In adults who are unoperated or previously palliated, morbidity and mortality is high. Late repair should be considered to improve outcome.

Late complications in repaired patients include:

Pulmonary regurgitation: (especially if previously placed transannular patch). This can lead to right ventricular dilatation and systolic dysfunction. It is a major clinical concern, particularly with regard to timing of reintervention.

Right ventricular outflow tract aneurysmal dilatation.

Tricuspid regurgitation: secondary to right ventricle dilatation.

Aortic regurgitation +/− aortic root dilatation is described.

Residual right ventricular outflow tract obstruction.

Residual VSD.

Endocarditis.

Tendency to atrial arrhythmias.

Ventricular arrhythmia: the usual focus is the RVOT. Increased QRS duration > 180 ms is a marker for sustained VT and sudden cardiac death.

Late sudden death, presumably arrhythmic, is recognized.

Transposition of the great arteries (D-transposition of the great arteries)

There is ventriculoarterial *discordance* and atrioventricular *concordance*: the aorta arises discordantly from the morphological right ventricle and the pulmonary artery arises discordantly from the morphological left ventricle. The atria connect concordantly to the ventricles (right atrium to right ventricle and left atrium to left ventricle). The aorta sits to the right and anterior to the pulmonary trunk (dextro-transposition or D-transposition).

Survival depends upon a connection allowing mixing which may be provided by a patent ductus arteriosus and patent foramen ovale or associated ventricular septal defect.

Presentation

Usually born at term with the clinical course largely determined by associated anomalies and degree of mixing between systemic and pulmonary circulations. Approximately 1/3 of patients have associated anomalies, which typically include VSD and pulmonary stenosis (*left ventricular outflow tract obstruction*).

Initial management in neonates may involve prostaglandin E1 infusion to maintain patency of the ductus arteriosus and balloon atrial septostomy (Rashkind procedure), which can be performed percutaneously under echocardiographic/angiographic guidance.

Subsequent surgical strategies

1. Atrial switch. Mustard and Senning procedures. Largely replaced by the arterial switch procedure. A conduit or 'baffle' is formed following excision of the interatrial septum to divert systemic venous return to the left ventricle via the mitral valve and pulmonary venous return to the right ventricle via the tricuspid valve. The right ventricle functions as the systemic ventricle.
2. Arterial switch. The aorta and pulmonary artery are repositioned correctly. The coronary arteries are re-anastomosed. Can be performed in the first two weeks of life. The left ventricle functions as the systemic ventricle.

3. Rastelli procedure (TGA + large VSD + pulmonary stenosis). Closure of VSD and formation of conduit from the right ventricle to pulmonary artery. Patch placed obstructing flow from the right ventricle to aorta. The left ventricle functions as the systemic ventricle. May be performed after an early palliation, e.g. modified Blalock-Taussig shunt.

Long term complications

1. Atrial switch: (the previous intervention in most current adults with TGA), failure of morphologic right ventricle (supporting systemic circulation), systemic AV valve regurgitation, arrhythmia (including sinus node dysfunction and intra-atrial re-entrant tachycardia), sudden cardiac death (likely arrhythmic), baffle leak or obstruction.
2. Arterial switch: right ventricular outflow tract obstruction, neoaortic valve regurgitation, neoaortic root dilatation, coronary obstruction.
3. Rastelli: conduit obstruction, subaortic stenosis (LV–aorta tunnel), arrhythmia, sudden cardiac death (likely arrhythmic), left ventricular dysfunction.

Congenitally corrected transposition of the great arteries (L-transposition of the great arteries)

Characterized by both ventriculoarterial and atrioventricular discordance, or 'double discordance'. As a result, the morphologic right ventricle supports the systemic circulation. The aorta sits anteriorly and to the left of the pulmonary artery (levo-transposition or L-transposition).

Usually has associated lesions which contribute to the presentation, typically: VSD, pulmonary stenosis and systemic AV valve abnormalities.

Clinical features

Right heart failure (systemic ventricle)
Tricuspid regurgitation (systemic AV valve)
Cyanosis can occur if associated lesions present (VSD and significant pulmonary stenosis)
Conduction abnormalities: congenital and acquired complete heart block
May not be diagnosed until older adulthood, particularly in the absence of associated anomalies.

Management

Early palliation may be indicated (e.g. PA banding for large VSD, modified BT shunt for severe pulmonary stenosis).

Medical surveillance in some cases is the chosen strategy. Surgical repair, where indicated, may include the following:
Conventional or 'classic' repair is treatment of associated anomalies, typically: closure of the VSD, replacement of the systemic AV valve and relief of pulmonary stenosis. The latter may require formation of a valved conduit between the morphologic left ventricle and pulmonary artery.

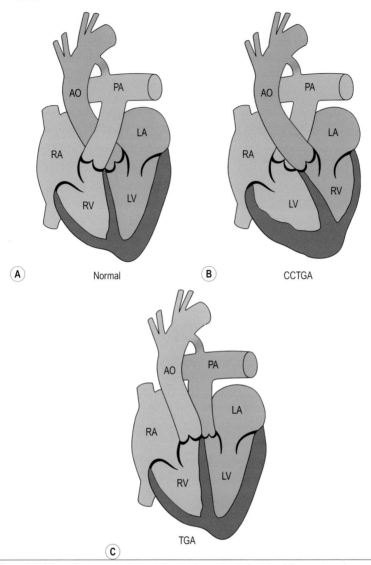

Figure 8.6 Schematic demonstrating variations in the anatomical origin of the great arteries. (A) Normal. (B) Congenitally corrected transposition of the great arteries (CCTGA). (C) Transposition of the great arteries (TGA).

The double-switch procedure, in which the morphologic left ventricle becomes the systemic ventricle, involves an atrial switch plus arterial switch or atrial switch with Rastelli procedure. The prerequisite is a morphologic left ventricle capable of supporting the systemic circulation and it may need to be 'trained' first with a pulmonary artery band. This is usually performed in childhood.

A Fontan-type repair may be considered if there is severe hypoplasia of either ventricle.

Heart transplantation may be offered in selected cases.

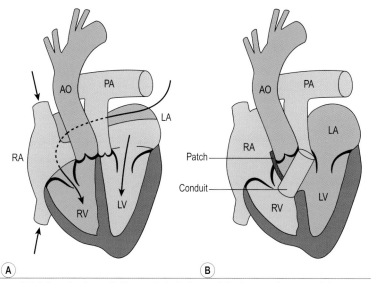

Figure 8.7 Schematic demonstrating anatomical changes following complex congenital cardiac surgery for transposition of the great arteries (TGA). (A) The Mustard/Senning operation for TGA. (B) The Rastelli operation for TGA and associated ventricular septal defect.

Cyanotic congenital heart disease

Cyanosis occurs in the presence of right to left shunting, with or without pulmonary hypertension.

Cyanotic conditions include transposition of the great arteries, tetralogy of Fallot, tricuspid atresia and Ebstein anomaly with ASD.

Eisenmenger syndrome describes a cyanotic condition of pulmonary vascular obstructive disease arising in the context of a pre-existing systemic-pulmonary vascular connection. Pulmonary hypertension results from progressive remodelling of the pulmonary vascular bed, with subsequent reversal of the left to right shunt or bidirectional shunting. Underlying conditions include VSD (Eisenmenger complex), PDA, ASD and atrioventricular septal defect. Iatrogenic causes include historically performed surgical procedures such as the Potts and Waterston shunts. Management of Eisenmenger syndrome is predominantly conservative.

There is a potential role for selective pulmonary vasodilators and some cases may be suitable for lung or heart–lung transplant.

Complications of cyanotic congenital heart disease include the following:
1. Secondary erythrocytosis: Due to chronic hypoxaemia. Hyperviscosity symptoms may be absent, even with very high haematocrit level. Venesection is generally contraindicated due to the increased stroke risk, particularly with concomitant iron deficiency. In emergencies it may be considered if Hb > 20 g/dl and Hct $> 65\%$ with iron and equal volume replacement.
2. Relative iron deficiency: The resulting microcytosis is associated with cerebrovascular events.
3. Bleeding and thrombosis: Coagulation and platelet abnormalities increase bleeding risks, such as pulmonary haemorrhage and perioperative bleeding. Thrombotic events may be associated with microcytosis, blood stasis, presence of prostheses and atrial arrhythmias. High risk of in situ pulmonary thrombus.
4. Cerebral abscess.
5. Paradoxical emboli
6. Hyperuricaemia.
7. Cholelithiasis.
8. Hypertrophic osteoarthropathy and scoliosis.

Univentricular physiology

The univentricular heart describes a functionally single ventricle which is not amenable to two-ventricle repair. Conditions with univentricular physiology include tricuspid atresia, hypoplastic left heart syndrome and double inlet left ventricle.

Tricuspid atresia (see Figure 8.8)

The tricuspid valve is not formed and there is an obligatory right to left shunt at atrial level.

Hypoplastic left heart

Spectrum of congenital cardiac anomalies characterized by underdevelopment of the left heart/ascending aorta. It is a prenatal/neonatal diagnosis and fatal without intervention.

Double inlet left ventricle

Usually the great vessels are transposed. The aortic arch is left-sided. Both atria are connected to the left ventricle. The right ventricle is rudimentary. A VSD is present.

The initial presentation and management of the functionally univentricular heart depend in part upon degree of pulmonary blood flow:
1. Associated pulmonary stenosis/atresia $\rightarrow$ reduced pulmonary blood flow and severe cyanosis.
   Requires a systemic to PA shunt.
2. No anatomic restriction to pulmonary flow $\rightarrow$ left to right shunting with features of congestive heart failure.
   Requires pulmonary artery banding.

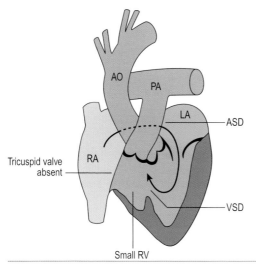

Figure 8.8 Schematic demonstrating the cardiac abnormalities in tricuspid atresia.

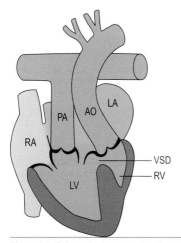

Figure 8.9 Schematic demonstrating the cardiac abnormalities in univentricular left heart physiology.

3. Rarely may be 'balanced' with a degree of pulmonary stenosis → mild cyanosis without congestive heart failure.
   No early intervention necessary.
   Further surgical palliation, usually in infancy when the PA pressure is low, is provided by the cavopulmonary shunt (Glenn procedure).

Some of these patients will undergo a Fontan operation in which caval blood is directed to the pulmonary arteries without circulating through a subpulmonary ventricle. Systemic to

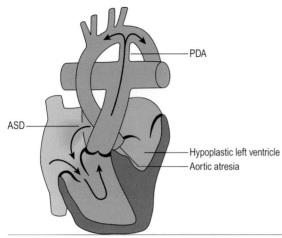

Figure 8.10 Schematic demonstrating cardiac abnormalities in hypoplastic left heart syndrome.

pulmonary flow is passive and driven by venous pressure. The circulation relies on good single ventricular function, lack of atrioventricular valve regurgitation and low pulmonary vascular resistance. Not all so-called Fontan circulations are identical as the term may be used to describe modifications of the original with different connections and materials.

In the original (atriopulmonary) Fontan procedure (first described for palliation of tricuspid atresia) the right atrium is directly anastomosed to the pulmonary artery. This leads in the long term to dilatation of the right atrium. This in turn can predispose to atrial arrhythmias, thrombus formation and pulmonary venous compression.

In the current era patients with univentricular physiology undergo total cavopulmonary connection (TCPC) surgery, usually in two stages: with a bidirectional Glenn followed by TCPC completion with either a lateral tunnel in the right atrium or more recently an extracardiac conduit. The TCPC may be fenestrated to create a small left-right shunt, intended to improve cardiac output and reduce excessive venous pressure. It is hoped that the modifications of the classic Fontan will reduce the problems associated with right atrial dilatation, though complications remain.

Complications of the Fontan/TCPC circulation

Characterized by low cardiac output, poor effort tolerance and chronic venous hypertension.

Issues:
Protein-losing enteropathy
Hepatic congestion
Progressive systemic ventricular dysfunction
Progressive AV valve incompetence
Right atrial enlargement (atriopulmonary Fontan)
Atrial arrhythmias common, poorly tolerated and increase in frequency over time
Sinus/AV node dysfunction common
Obstruction in circuit
Thromboembolism (sluggish flow, atrial arrhythmia, thrombophilic state). Can be pulmonary or systemic.

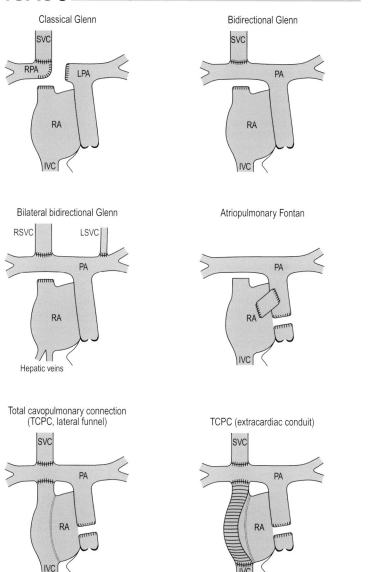

Figure 8.11 Schematic demonstrating variants of the Fontan operation. RPA: right pulmonary artery, LPA: left pulmonary artery, RA: right atrium, IVC: inferior vena cava, PA: pulmonary artery, RSVC: right superior vena cava, LSVC: left superior vena cava, TCPC: total cavopulmonary connection. Source: Adult congenital heart disease: a practical guide. Michael A. Gatzoulis, Lorna Swan, Judith Therrien, George Pantely, Eugene Braunwald. Blackwell Publishing, 2005.

Glossary of operations for congenital heart disease

Arterial switch (Jatene procedure)

Condition: Complete transposition of great arteries.
Purpose: Achievement of ventriculoarterial concordance (left ventricle to aorta and right ventricle to pulmonary artery), so that the left ventricle supports the systemic circulation.
Procedure: The great vessels are both transected above the valve level and each reattached to the contralateral ventricle. The coronary arteries are implanted with a surrounding button of aortic wall into the neoaorta.
Complications: Right ventricular outflow tract obstruction, neoaortic valve regurgitation, neoaortic root dilatation, coronary obstruction.

Atrial switch (see Mustard/Senning/procedure)

Blalock-Hanlon atrial septectomy

Condition: Transposition of great arteries.
Purpose: Mixing of blood at atrial level to improve arterial oxygen saturation.
Procedure: Palliative. Atrial septectomy perfomed surgically via right thoracotomy.
　　Superseded by the Rashkind procedure.

Blalock-Taussig shunt

Condition: Pulmonary stenosis, pulmonary atresia, tetralogy of Fallot.
Purpose: Increase pulmonary blood flow.
Procedure: Palliative. Anastomosis between subclavian artery and pulmonary artery.
Classic BT shunt: Direct end to side anastomosis. No longer performed.
Modified BT shunt: Interposition tube graft used.

Brock procedure

Condition: Tetralogy of Fallot.
Purpose: Increase pulmonary blood flow and reduce right to left shunting.
Procedure: Palliative. No longer performed. Resection of part of right infundibular tissue to reduce RV outflow tract obstruction.

Double switch procedure

Condition: Congenitally corrected transposition of great arteries.
Purpose: Anatomical correction of CCTGA so that the LV supports the systemic circulation.
　　May be preceded by pulmonary artery banding to 'train' the LV.
Procedure: Atrial switch with arterial switch or with Rastelli procedure.

Fontan procedure

Condition: Functionally univentricular heart.
Purpose: Final stage of palliation for functionally univentricular heart.
Procedure: Systemic venous return is directed to the pulmonary artery and relies on passive flow. Systemic and pulmonary circulations are separated but a fenestration may be placed to allow left to right shunting and reduce pressure in the circuit. Many variations. Currently used is the total cavopulmonary connection (TCPC).

Glenn shunt

Condition: Cyanotic congenital heart disease.

Purpose: Increase pulmonary blood flow.

Procedure: Palliative. Cavopulmonary shunt. Does not cause extra volume overload of the systemic ventricle (unlike arteriopulmonary shunts). Prerequisite of low pulmonary vascular resistance.

- Classic Glenn: SVC to right pulmonary artery. Right pulmonary artery separated from main pulmonary artery. No longer used. Commonly complicated by development of pulmonary arteriovenous malformations.
- Bidirectional Glenn: SVC to right pulmonary artery, which remains in continuity with the main pulmonary artery.

Mustard procedure/Senning procedure/atrial switch

Condition: Transposition of great arteries.

Purpose: Directs systemic venous return to the pulmonary circulation and pulmonary venous blood to the systemic circulation.

Procedure: Atrial switch. In the Mustard procedure, the baffle is made from pericardium or synthetic material. In the Senning procedure, atrial tissue is used to create the baffle.

Complications: Systemic right ventricular failure, systemic atrioventricular valve regurgitation, arrhythmia, sudden death, baffle leak or obstruction.

Potts shunt

Condition: Congenital heart disease with restricted pulmonary blood flow. Pulmonary stenosis/pulmonary atresia.

Purpose: Increase pulmonary blood flow.

Procedure: Direct anastomosis between left pulmonary artery and descending aorta. No longer performed.

Complications: Pulmonary hypertension, LV volume overload, left pulmonary artery distortion.

Pulmonary artery banding

Condition: Multiple.

Purpose: Protect lungs from high pulmonary blood flow or to train the subpulmonary ventricle to function as a systemic ventricle.

Procedure: Intentional pulmonary stenosis.

Rashkind procedure

Condition: Complete transposition of the great arteries.

Purpose: Mixing of blood at atrial level to improve arterial oxygen saturation and buys time prior to definitive surgery.

Procedure: Balloon atrial septostomy. Palliative catheter-based procedure.

Rastelli procedure

Condition: Complete transposition of the great arteries with VSD and pulmonary outflow tract obstruction.

Purpose: The LV supports the systemic circulation.

Procedure: The VSD is closed with a patch that connects the LV to the aorta. The pulmonary artery is separated from the annulus, the annulus is oversewn and a valved conduit is placed between the RV and pulmonary artery.

Ross procedure

Condition: Aortic valve disease.

Purpose: Relieve LVOTO.

Procedure: Native pulmonary valve, annulus and root moved to the aortic position (aortic autograft). The RVOT is reconstructed using a pulmonary homograft conduit.

Senning procedure: (see Mustard/Senning procedure)

Waterston shunt

Condition: Congenital heart disease with restricted pulmonary blood flow. Pulmonary stenosis/pulmonary atresia.

Purpose: Increase pulmonary blood flow.

Procedure: Palliative. Direct anastomosis between right pulmonary artery and ascending aorta. No longer performed.

Complications: Pulmonary hypertension, LV volume overload, right pulmonary artery distortion.

TOPIC **9**

Pulmonary vascular disorders

Topic Contents

Pulmonary hypertension

Definition

Mean pulmonary artery pressure (PAP):
> 25 mmHg at rest
> 30 mmHg with exercise.

Incidence

Estimated at 500–1000 new cases annually
Approximately 2–3 per million per year with a prevalence of 15 per million
Occurs in men, women and children of all ages
Most common in females between 20 and 40 years old (M:F 1:2)
Rare in children, but sometimes seen in infants born with valvular defects.

Causes and Classification (ESC Guidelines 2004)

1. Pulmonary arterial hypertension (PAH)
    1.1. Idiopathic pulmonary arterial hypertension (IPAH)
    1.2. Familial pulmonary arterial hypertension (FPAH)
    1.3. Associated with APAH
        1.3.1. Connective tissue disease
        1.3.2. Congenital systemic to pulmonary shunts
        1.3.3. Portal hypertension
        1.3.4. HIV infection
        1.3.5. Drugs and toxins
        1.3.6. Other

1.4. Associated with significant venous or capillary involvement
    1.4.1. Pulmonary veno-occlusive disease (PVOD)
    1.4.2. Pulmonary capillary haemangiomatosis
1.5. Persistent pulmonary hypertension of the newborn (PPHN)
2. Pulmonary hypertension associated with left heart disease
    2.1. Left-sided atrial or ventricular heart disease
    2.2. Left-sided valvular heart disease
3. Pulmonary hypertension associated with lung respiratory disease/hypoxia
    3.1. Chronic obstructive pulmonary disease
    3.2. Interstitial lung disease
    3.3. Sleep disordered breathing
    3.4. Alveolar hypoventilation disorders
    3.5. Chronic exposure to high altitude
    3.6. Developmental abnormalities
4. Pulmonary hypertension due to chronic thrombotic and/or embolic disease
    4.1. Thromboembolic obstruction of proximal pulmonary arteries
    4.2. Thromboembolic obstruction of distal pulmonary arteries
    4.3. Non-thrombotic pulmonary embolism (tumour, foreign material)
5. Miscellaneous (sarcoid, histiocytosis X)

Investigations

Electrocardiogram
Nocturnal oxygen saturation ($>96\%$)
Chest radiograph
Respiratory function tests
Echocardiogram
Ventilation perfusion scan
High-resolution CT scan
Helical CT with pulmonary angiography
Blood tests
Haematology
    Full blood count
    ESR
    Clotting screen
    Thrombophilia screen
    Protein C
    Protein S
    Lupus anticoagulant
    Antithrombin III
    Leiden factor V
    Abnormal haemoglobin
    Blood group
Biochemistry
    Urea and electrolytes
    Liver function tests
    CRP
    Serum ACE
    Thyroid function
    Arterial blood gases
    Autoimmune screen
    Anti-nuclear factor
    Anti-smooth muscle

Anti-centromere
Anti-SCL70
Anti-RNP
Anti-phospholipid
Anti-mitochondria
Anti-parietal
Microbiology
Hepatitis B status
Hepatitis C status
VDRL/TPHA
HIV
Viral titres
CMV, EBV
H simplex
Toxoplasma, Pneumocystis
Aspergillus screen
Right heart catheterization (see Chapter 5 for normal chamber pressures)
Right artial pressure
Pulmonary arterial pressure (systolic, diastolic and mean)
Pulmonary capillary wedge pressure
Cardiac output (thermodilution or Fick methods)
Systemic vascular resistance
Arterial and mixed venous oxygen saturation
Acute vasodilator testing

Commonly used vaso-active dugs for vasodilator study drug

Table 9.1 Commonly used vaso-active dugs for vasodilator study					
Drug	Route	Half-life	Dose range[a]	Increments[b]	Duration[c]
Epoprostenol	Intravenous	3 min	2–12 ng/kg/min	2 ng/kg/min	10 min
Adenosine	Intravenous	5–10 s	50–350 μg/kg/min	50 μg/kg/min	2 min
Nitric oxide	Inhaled	15–30 s	10–20 ppm	–	5 min[d]

[a]Initial dose and maximal dose suggested.
[b]Increments of dose by each step.
[c]Duration of administration on each step.
[d]For NO a single step with the dose range is suggested.

Algorithm for investigation suspected pulmonary hypertension (Figure 9.1)

Management

Anticoagulants
Diuretics
Calcium channel blockers
Endothelin receptor antagonist
Prostacyclin
Oxygen
Transplantation

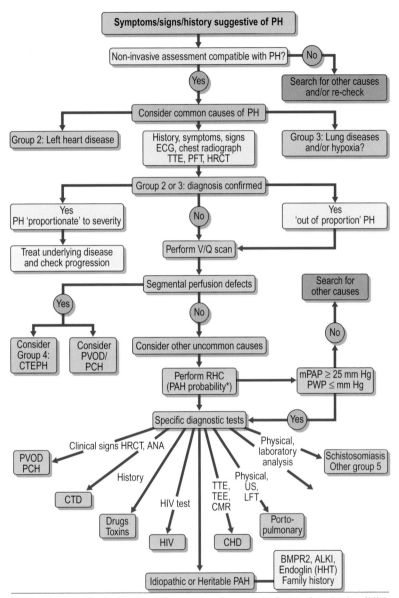

Figure 9.1 Diagnostic algorithm for the investigation of suspected pulmonary hypertension. ALK-1, activin-receptor-like kinase; ANA, anti-nuclear antibodies; BMPR2, bone morphogenetic protein receptor 2; CHD, congenital heart disease; CMR, cardiac magnetic resonance; CTD, connective tissue disease; Group, clinical group; HHT, hereditary haemorrhagic telangiectasia; HIV, human immunodeficiency virus; HRCT, high-resolution computed tomography; LFT, liver

Pulmonary thromboembolism

Risk factors

1. Major risk factors (relative risk 5–20):
   a. Surgery*
      Major abdominal/pelvic surgery
      Hip/knee replacement
      Postoperative intensive care
   b. Obstetrics
      Late pregnancy
      Caesarean section
      Puerperium
   c. Lower limb problems
      Fracture
      Varicose veins
   d. Malignancy
      Abdominal/pelvic
      Advanced/metastatic
   e. Reduced mobility
      Hospitalization
      Institutional care
   f. Miscellaneous
      Previous proven VTE
2. Minor risk factors (relative risk 2–4):
   a. Cardiovascular
      Congenital heart disease
      Congestive cardiac failure
      Hypertension
      Superficial venous thrombosis
      Indwelling central vein catheter
   b. Oestrogens
      Oral contraceptive
      Hormone replacement therapy
3. Miscellaneous
   COPD
   Neurological disability
   Occult malignancy
   Thrombotic disorders
   Long-distance sedentary travel
   Obesity
   Other (inflammatory bowel disease, nephrotic syndrome, chronic dialysis,
      myeloproliferative disorders, paroxysmal nocturnal haemoglobinuria).

---

function tests; mPAP, mean pulmonary arterial pressure; PAH, pulmonary arterial hypertension; PCH, pulmonary capillary haemangiomatosis; PFT, pulmonary function test; PH, pulmonary hypertension; PVOD, pulmonary veno-occlusive disease; PWP, pulmonary wedge pressure; RHC, right heart catheterization; TEE, transoesophageal echocardiography; TTE, transthoracic echocardiography; US, ultrasonography; V/Q, ventilation/perfusion lung scan. Adapted with permission from European Heart Journal 2009; 30: 2493–2537.

Investigations (Figure 9.2)

Chest X ray
D-dimer – normal range 0–218 ng/ml
CT pulmonary angiogram
Isotope lung scan if CTPA unavailable or equivoval
Lower limb ultrasound if indicated

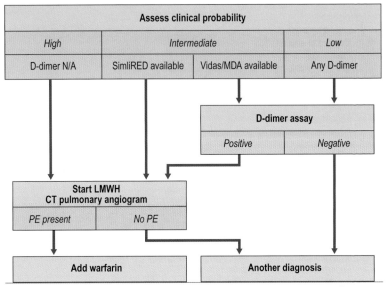

Figure 9.2 Investigation and treatment algorithm for management of pulmonary emboli.

Treatment

Thrombolysis (alteplase 50 mg) in massive PE
Heparin (low-molecular-weight or unfractionated if reversal a possibility)
Oral anticoagulation (at least 6 months)

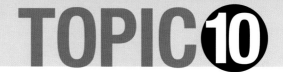

Systemic vascular disease

Topic Contents

Aortic wall thickness

Measurement of aortic wall thickness can be used to assess cardiovascular risk. Aortic mean average wall thickness is increased by atheromatous disease which preferentially affects the aortic media. Aortic mean average wall thickness also increases with age, is higher in males and non-Caucasian races.
Men: mean average wall thickness 2.32 mm
Women: mean average wall thickness 2.11 mm.

Aortic dissection

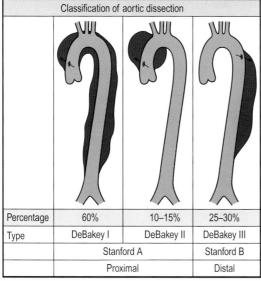

Classification of aortic dissection		
Percentage	60%	10–15%	25–30%
Type	DeBakey I	DeBakey II	DeBakey III
	Stanford A		Stanford B
	Proximal		Distal

Figure 10.1 Anatomical classification of thoracic aortic dissection.

Classification

DeBakey

Type 1 Involvement of ascending and descending aorta with extensive distal extension.
Type 2 Involvement restricted to ascending aorta. Typically seen in Marfan's syndrome.
Type 3 Involvement restricted to descending aorta, distal to left subclavian artery.

Stanford classification

Type A (proximal) Involvement of ascending aorta (DeBakey types 1 & 2)
Type B (distal) No involvement of ascending aorta (DeBakey type 3).

Secondary hypertension

Table 10.1 **Anatomical classification of thoracic aortic dissection**

Causes	Marker	Normal range
Kidney disease	Blood	
Creatinine	Men:	45–90 µmol/L (0.5–1.0 mg/dl)
	Women:	60–110 µmol/L (0.7–1.2 mg/dl)
Urine output		
GFR	Men:	< 70 ml/min/m^2
	Women:	< 60 ml/min/m^2
Cushing's syndrome	Dexamethasone suppression test	
Cortisol	N/A	
ACTH	N/A	
Phaeochromocytoma	24-hour urine	
	Epinephrine	0.5–20 µg/24 hours
	Norenephrine	15–80 µg/24 hours
	Dopamine	65–400 µg/24 hours
	Renin	20–100 mU/L
Conn's syndrome	Low renin	<20
	Aldosterone/renin ratio	>750
Hyperthyroidism	TSH	0.3–3.0 mIU/L
	Thyroxine (T4)	4–11 µg/dl
	T3	130–220 ng/dl

GFR = glomerular filtration rate, ACTH = adrenocorticotrophic hormone, TSH = thyroid stimulation hormone.

Appendix 1

Cardiac pharmacology

Class	Name	Dose	Frequency	Blood levels	Special considerations
Cardiac glycosides	Digoxin	Loading 500 mg 2–3 doses IV or orally Maintenance 62.5–500 mg	OD	0.8–2.0 ng/ml	Blood level sampling must be >8 hours post last oral dose
Betablockers	Propranolol	40–160 mg	BD-TDS		
	Atenolol	50–100 mg	OD		
	Bisoprolol	1.25–10 mg	OD		
	Carvedilol	3.125–25 mg	BD		
	Esmolol	50–200 µg/kg/min IV			
	Labetalol	50–800mg PO, 50 mg IV injection, 2 mg/min IV infusion	BD		
	Metoprolol	50–100 mg 5 mg IV every 5 min up to 15 mg max	TDS		
	Nebivolol	1.25–10 mg	OD		
	Sotalol	40–160 mg	BD		
ACE inhibitors	Captopril	6.25–25 mg	TDS		
	Enalapril	2.5–20 mg	OD		
	Fosinopril	10–40 mg	OD		
	Lisinopril	2.5–20 mg	OD		
	Perindopril	2–8 mg	OD		
	Ramipril	1.25–10 mg	OD		
	Trandolapril	0.5–4 mg	OD		
Angiotensin II receptor antagonists	Candesartan	4–16 mg	OD		
	Irbesartan	75–300 mg	OD		
	Losartan	50–100 mg	OD		
	Telmisartan	40–80 mg	OD		
	Valsartan	80–160 mg	OD		
Direct renin inhibitors	Aliskiren	150–300 mg	OD		

Class	Name	Dose	Frequency	Blood levels	Special considerations
Nitrates	Glyceryl trinitrate	0.3–1 mg sl 10–200 μg/ min IV	PRN		Nitrate free period (8+ h/ day) required to prevent tachyphylaxis
	Isosorbide dinitrate	30–120 mg	BD		
	Isosorbide mononitrate	20–60 mg	BD		
	Isosorbide mononitrate modified release	30–120 mg	OD		
Calcium channel blockers	Verapamil	40–120 mg 0.1 mg/kg	TDS IV Bolus		
	Diltiazem	60–120 mg	TDS		
	Amlodipine	5–10 mg	OD		
	Felodipine	5–20 mg	OD		
	Lercanidipine	10–20 mg	OD		
	Nifedipine	5–20 mg	TDS		
Potassium channel activators	Nicorandil	10–30 mg	BD		
Positive inotropes	Dobutamine	2.5–10 μg/kg/ min	IV Infusion		
	Dopamine	2–10 μg/kg/min	IV Infusion		
	Dopexamine	0.5–6 μg/kg/min	IV Infusion		
	Isoprenaline	0.5–20 μg/min	IV Infusion		
	Norepinephrine	0.02–1.5 mcg/ kg/min	IV Infusion		
	Epinephrine	0.02–1.0 mcg/ kg/min	IV Infusion		
	Milrinone	50 μg/kg loading over 10 mins 375–750 ng/ kg/min	IV Infusion		
	Enoximone	90 μg/kg/min for 10–30 min loading, followed by 5–20 μg/kg/ min maintenance			*
	Levosimendan	12 μg/kg bolus + 24 h 0.1–0.2 μg/ kg/min infusion	IV Infusion		* Initial trials used bolus for loading. Now recommended to start infusion without loading bolus.

Diuretics	Bendroflumethiazide	2.5–5.0 mg	OD	
	Chlorthalidone	25–200 mg	OD	
	Cyclopenthiazide	250–500 μg	OD	
	Indapamide	2.5 mg	OD	
	Metolazone	2.5–40 mg	OD	
	Furosemide	20–160 mg po 250 mg loading, 10–20 mg/h IV	OD-BD IV infusion	
	Bumetanide	1–5 mg	OD	
	Amiloride	5–20 mg	OD	
	Spironolactone	25–400 mg	OD	
	Eplerenone	25–50 mg	OD	
	Mannitol	50–200 g IV	IV infusion over 24 hours	
	Nesiritide	0.3–0.6 μg/kg bolus + 0.015–0.03 μg/kg/min infusion		*
Fast Na^+ channel blockers	Disopyramide	100–300 mg	TDS	
	Flecainide	PO 50–200 mg IV 2 mg/kg over 30 min, max 150 mg	BD	
	Lignocaine/ Lidocaine	IV bolus 50–100 mg infusion 4 mg/min first 30 min, then 2 mg/min next 2 hours, then 1 mg/min maintenance		
	Mexilitine	PO loading 400–600 mg Maintenance 200–250 mg	TDS-QDS	
	Procainamide	IV infusion Loading 500–600 mg over 30 min 2–6 mg/min maintenance		
	Propafenone	150–300 mg	TDS	
	Quinidine	200–400 mg	TDS	

APPENDIX 1

Class	Name	Dose	Frequency	Blood levels	Special considerations
SA Node I$_f$ blocker	Ivabradine	2.5–7.5 mg	BD		
Late Na$^+$ channel blocker	Ranolazine	500–1000 mg	BD		
Adenosine agonist	Adenosine	3–24 mg	IV		Bolus via large peripheral vein with 10–20 ml flush
Potassium channel blockers	Amiodarone	PO Loading 200 mg TDS for week 1, 200 mg BD for week 2 Maintenance 200 mg OD IV 5 mg/kg over 1 hour	PO IV		
	Dronedarone	400 mg	BD	*	
	Bretylium	IV Loading 5–10 mg/kg over 10–30 min Maintenance 1–2 mg/min infusion	IV		
Vasodilators	Hydralazine	PO 25–50 mg IV Infusion Loading 200–300 μg/min for 1 hour Maintenance 50–150 μg/min	PO BD IV		
	Minoxidil	2.5–25 mg	BD		
	Sodium Nitroprusside	0.5–1.5 μg/kg/min	IV Infusion		
Alpha adrenoceptor blockers	Doxazosin	1–16 mg	OD		
	Indoramin	25–100 mg	BD		
	Prazosin	0.5–5 mg	BD-TDS		

	Phenoxybenzamine	IV 1 mg/kg over 2 hours	OD	Daily dose
	Phentolamine	IV 2–5 mg	PRN	
Centrally acting antihypertensives	Clonidine	50–400 µg	TDS	
	Methyldopa	250 mg–1 g	TDS	
	Moxonidine	200 µg OD– 300 µg BD	OD-BD	
Metabolic manipulators	Perhexiline	100 mg	BD	*
	Trimetazidine	20 mg	TDS	*
Anticoagulants	Heparin	5000– 10 000 Units IV loading bolus followed by 15–25 U/kg/h infusion		
	Low-molecular- weight heparin: Dalteparin	Prophylaxis 2500 U Treatment 7500–18000 U/day	OD-BD	Dose is weight determined: <46 kg, 46–56 kg, 57–68 kg, 69–82 kg, >83 kg
	Low-molecular- weight heparin: Enoxaparin	Prophylaxis 20–40 mg Treatment PE/DVT 1.5 mg/kg ACS 1 mg/kg	OD OD BD	
	Low-molecular- weight heparin: Tinzaparin	Prophylaxis 3500 U (low risk)–50 U/kg (high risk) Treatment 175 U/kg	OD	
	Bilvalirudin	750 µg/kg IV Loading, then 1.75 mg/kg/h for 4 h		*
	Warfarin			
Antiplatelet agents	Aspirin	75–300 mg	OD	
	Clopidogrel	300–600 mg Loading 75 mg maintenance	OD	

APPENDIX 1

Class	Name	Dose	Frequency	Blood levels	Special considerations
	Prasugrel	60 mg loading 10 mg maintenance	OD		
	Dipyrimadole	100–200 mg	BD		
	Abciximab	250 µg/kg IV loading, then 125 ng/kg/min		Max 10 µg/ min	
	Eptifibatide	180 µg/kg IV loading, then 2 µg/kg/min IV infusion			
	Tirofiban	400 ng/kg/min IV loading for 30 min, then 100 ng/kg/min maintenance			
Fibrinolytics	Alteplase	15 mg IV injection, then 50 mg IV over 30 min, then 35 mg IV over 60 min			
	Reteplase	10 Units bolus followed by 10 Units 30 min later			
	Streptokinase	1.5 million Units over 60 min (MI), 250 000 Units over 30 min (PE)			
	Tenecteplase	0.5 mg/kg IV bolus		Max 50 mg	
Hemostatics	Protamine	25–50 mg IV infusion at 2.5–5 mg/min			
	Aprotinin	Loading dose 1–2 Million Units, maintenance IV infusion 250–500,000 units/hr			Only licensed for use during cardiac surgery
	Tranexamic acid	1–1.5 g	BD-TDS		
Prostaglandins	Epoprostenol	2–12 ng/kg/min IV infusion			
	Iloprost	2.5–5 µg Nebulized	6–9x/day		

Endothelin antagonists	Bosentan	62.5–250 mg	BD		
	Sitaxentan	100 mg	OD	*	
PDE5 inhibitors	Sildenafil	20 mg	TDS		
Statins	Atorvastatin	10–80 mg	Nocte		
	Pravastatin	10–40 mg	Nocte		
	Rosuvastatin	5–20 mg	Nocte		Elderly and Asians sensitive – starting dose 5 mg
	Simvastatin	10–80 mg	Nocte		
Nicotinic acid	Nicotinic acid	375 mg–2 g	Nocte		
Cholesterol absorption inhibitor	Ezetimibe	10 mg	OD		
Fibrates	Bezafibrate	200 mg	TDS		
	Fenofibrate	200 mg	OD		
	Gemfibrozil	300–600 mg	BD		
Fatty acids	Omega-3	1–4 g	OD		

*Not licensed in the United Kingdom at the time of writing.

Appendix 2

United Kingdom Department of Vehicle Licensing and Transport Regulations (Revised November 2008) Crown copyright

Condition	Private License (Group 1)	Heavy Goods Vehicle (HGV) License (Group 2)
Stable angina	Stable symptoms No notification required	Notification required License revoked. Relicensing if: Symptom free for 6 weeks, and functional stress test demonstrates lack of inducible cardiac ischaemia
Unstable angina and acute coronary syndromes	1. One week post successful coronary angioplasty/stent, providing LVEF > 40% 2. Four weeks if no revascularization/ unsuccessful angioplasty/ stent	Disqualification for 6 weeks. Relicensing if symptom free and functional stress test demonstrates lack of inducible cardiac ischaemia
Elective PCI	One week	Disqualification for 6 weeks. Relicensing if symptom free and functional stress test demonstrates lack of inducible cardiac ischaemia
CABG surgery	Four weeks	Disqualification for 3 months. Relicensing if symptom free, LVEF > 40% and functional stress test demonstrates lack of inducible cardiac ischaemia
Left ventricular impairment		LVEF <40% – Bar to holding Group 2 license
Arrhythmia sinus arrhythmias, AF, atrial flutter, SVT, VT, AV conduction delays	Driving must cease if arrhythmia has caused, or is likely to cause, incapacity. Recommence driving once arrhythmia treated and controlled for 4 weeks	Disqualification if arrhythmia has caused, or is likely to cause, incapacity. Relicensing if arrhythmia controlled for 3 months without incapacity

Successful catheter ablation	Two days	Driving cease for: 6 weeks if arrhythmia likely to cause incapacity 2 weeks if arrhythmia unlikely to cause incapacity
Pacemaker implantation (including box change)	One week	6 weeks
Unpaced congenital complete heart block	May drive if asymptomatic	Disqualification
Implantable cardiodefibrillator (ICD)	Driving disallowed for: 6 months following implantation 6 months following shock or symptomatic ATP 2 years if shock/ATP accompanied by incapacity (unless inappropriate shock (4 weeks) or new antiarrhythmic strategy and asymptomatic (6 months)	Disqualification
ICD box change	One week	N/A
ICD lead change/reposition	One month	
ICD for primary prevention	One month post implantation	
ICD for stable VT without incapacity	One month post implantation if: LVEF>35% VT without fast cycle length (RR <250 ms) VT terminated by ATP without acceleration to RR <250 ms	
Thoracic or abdominal aortic aneurysm	Inform DVLA if aortic diameter >6 cm Annual review re fitness to drive, if BP controlled and aneurysm not enlarging. Disqualification if aortic diameter >6.5 cm	Disqualification if aortic diameter >5.5 cm
Chronic aortic dissection	Continue providing satisfactory BP control	May continue to drive providing: A. Maximum aortic diameter (including false lumen) <5.5 cm B. Complete thrombosis of false lumen C. BP well controlled
Hypertension	None	Disqualification is systolic BP >180 mmHg or diastolic BP >100 mmHg

Condition	Private License (Group 1)	Heavy Goods Vehicle (HGV) License (Group 2)
Hypertrophic cardiomyopathy		Disqualification if symptomatic. Licensing if 3 of following criteria are met: No family history of SCD LV wall $<$3 mm thick No VT $>$25 mmHg increase in BP with exercise
Dilated cardiomyopathy		Disqualification if symptomatic
Arrhythmogenic right ventricular dysplasia	Disqualification if arrhythmia leads to incapacity	Disqualification if symptomatic. Specialist electrophysiological assessment if asymptomatic
Heart failure	Driving allowed if no symptoms leading to incapacity	Disqualification if symptomatic or LVEF$<$ 40%
Left ventricular assist device	Disqualification at implantation. Reevaluation at 6 months post implantation	Disqualification permanent
Heart transplantation		Disqualification if symptomatic. If asymptomatic, driver must: Pass exercise test LVEF $>$40% No other disqualifying conditions
Heart valve disease, including valve surgery		Disqualification if: Symptomatic Cerebral embolism within 12 months
Congenital heart disease	Driving allowed. Medical review annually if complex or severe disease	Disqualification if complex or severe disorder is present
Syncope: Vasovagal syncope/ simple faint	No driving restrictions	No driving restrictions
Syncope: Cardiac or neurological risk factors/ abnormalities and low risk of recurrence	4 weeks after cause identified/ treated	3 months after cause identified/ treated
Syncope: Cardiac risk factors/ abnormalities and/or high risk of recurrence	4 weeks after cause identified/ treated 6 months if no cause identified/ treated	3 months after cause identified/ treated 12 months if no cause identified/treated

Syncope: No risk factors/ abnormalities identified	6 months	12 months
ECG abnormality: previous MI		Driver must pass functional testing
ECG abnormality: LBBB		Driver must pass functional testing
ECG abnormality: Pre-excitation		Can be ignored unless associated with arrhythmia

Appendix 3

Bibliography

Topic 1

Angelini P: Coronary artery anomalies – current clinical issues: definitions, classification, incidence, relevance and treatment guidelines, *Texas Heart Inst J* 29(4):271–278, 2002.

Basso C, Maron BJ, Corrado D, et al: Clinical profile of congenital coronary artery anomalies with origin from the wrong aortic sinus leading to sudden death in young competitive athletes, *JACC* 35(6):1493–1501, 2000.

Davies JE, Whinnett ZI, Francis DP: Evidence of a dominant backward-propagating "suction" wave responsible for diastolic coronary filling in humans, attenuated in left ventricular hypertrophy, *Circulation* 113:1768–1778, 2006.

Fuster V, O'Rourke RA, Walsh RA, Poole-Wilson P, editors: *Hurst's The Heart*, ed 12, 2008, McGraw-Hill.

Topic 2

Cerqueira MD, Weissman NJ, Dilsizian V, et al: Standardised myocardial segmentation and nomenclature for tomography imaging of the heart. Scientific statement from the AHA writing group on myocardial segmentation and registration for cardiac imaging, *Circulation* 105:539, 2002.

Gibbons RJ, Balady GJ, Bricker JT, et al: ACC/AHA 2002 guideline update for exercise testing: summary article: a report of the American College of Cardiology/American Heart Association Task Force on Practice Guidelines (Committee to Update the 1997 Exercise Testing Guidelines), *Circulation* 106:1883, 2002.

Kern MJ, Lerman A, Bech JW, et al: Physiological assessment of coronary artery disease in the cardiac catheterization laboratory. A scientific statement from the American Heart Association Committee on Diagnostic and Interventional Cardiac Catheterization, Council on Clinical Cardiology, *Circulation* 114:1321–1341, 2006.

Klocke FJ, Baird MJ, Lorell BH, et al: ACC/AHA/ASNC guidelines for the clinical use of cardiac radionuclide imaging–executive summary: a report of the American College of Cardiology/American Heart Association Task Force on Practice Guidelines (ACC/AHA/ASNC Committee to Revise the 1995 Guidelines for the Clinical Use of Cardiac Radionuclide Imaging), *J Am Coll Cardiol* 42:1318, 2003.

Pijls NH, De Bruyne B: Coronary pressure measurement and fractional flow reserve, *Heart* 80:539–542, 1998.

Universal definition of myocardial infarction. Joint ESC/ACCF/AHA/WHF Task Force for the Redefinition of Myocardial Infarction, *Circulation* 116(22):2634–2653, 2007.

Topic 3

Graham I, Atar D, Borch-Johnsen K, et al: European guidelines on cardiovascular disease prevention in clinical practice: full text. Fourth Joint Task Force of the European Society of Cardiology and other societies on cardiovascular disease prevention in clinical practice, *Eur J Cardiovasc Prev Rehabil* 14(Suppl 2):S1–S113, 2007.

Rosenson RS, Koenig W: Utility of inflammatory markers in the management of coronary artery disease, *Am J Cardiol* 92:10i–18i, 2003.

Rydén L, Standl E, Bartnik M, et al: Guidelines on diabetes, pre-diabetes, and cardiovascular diseases: executive summary. The Task Force on Diabetes and Cardiovascular Diseases of the European Society of Cardiology (ESC) and of the European Association for the Study of Diabetes (EASD), *Eur Heart J* 28:88–136, 2007.

Topic 4

Albrecht P, Arnold J, Krishnamachari S, et al: Exercise recordings for the detection of T wave alternans. Promises and pitfalls, *J Electrocardiol* 29(Suppl):46–51, 1996.

Braunwald's Heart Disease: *A textbook of cardiovascular medicine*, ed 7, Elsevier.

Josephson MJ: *Clinical Cardiac Electrophysiology: Techniques and Interpretations*, ed 4, Lippincott Williams & Wilkins.

Marcus FI, Zareba W, Sherrill D, et al: Evaluation of the normal values for signal-averaged electrocardiogram, *J Cardiovasc Electrophysiol* 18(2):231–233, 2007.

Rautaharju PM, Surawicz B, Gettes LS, et al: AHA/ACCF/HRS recommendations for the standardization and interpretation of the electrocardiogram: Part IV: The ST segment, T and U waves, and the QT interval, *Circulation* 119:241–250, 2009.

Zipes DP, Jalife J: *Cardiac Electrophysiology from Cell to Bedside*, ed 4, WB Saunders.

Topic 5

ACC/AHA: 2005 Guideline update for the diagnosis and management of chronic heart failure in the adult, *Circulation* 112:154–235, 2005.

ACC/AHA guidelines for the evaluation and management of chronic heart failure in the adult, *Circulation* 104:2996–3007, 2001.

Braunwald's Heart Disease: *A textbook of cardiovascular medicine*, ed 7, Elsevier.

British Society of Echocardiography Education Committee: Guidelines for Chamber Quantification.

De Lemos JA, McGuire DK, Drazner MH: B-type natriuretic peptide in cardiovascular disease, *Lancet* 362:316–322, 2003.

ESC Guidelines for the diagnosis and treatment of acute and chronic heart failure 2008, *EHJ* 29:2388–2442, 2008.

Klein AL, Garcia MJ, editors: *Diastology – Clinical Approach to Diastolic Heart Failure*, Elsevier/Saunders.

Liu CP, Ting CT, Lawrence W, et al: Diminished contractile response to increased heart rate in intact human left ventricular hypertrophy. Systolic versus diastolic determinants, *Circulation* 88:1893–1906, 1993.

Maceira AM, Prasad SK, Khan M, et al: Normalized left ventricular systolic and diastolic function by steady state free precession cardiovascular magnetic resonance, *J Cardiovasc Magn Reson* 8:417–426, 2006.

Maceira AM, Prasad SK, Khan M, et al: Reference right ventricular systolic and diastolic function normalized to age, gender and body surface area from steady-state free precession cardiovascular magnetic resonance, *EHJ* 27:2879–2888, 2006.

Reynolds DW, Bartelt N, Taepke R, et al: Measurement of pulmonary artery diastolic pressure from the right ventricle, *JACC* 25:1176–1182, 1995.

Topic 6

ACC/AHA: 2006 Guidelines for the management of patients with valvular heart disease, *Circulation* 114:84–231, 2006.

British Society of Echocardiography Education Committee: Guidelines for Valve Quantification.

ESC Guidelines on the management of valvular heart disease, *Eur Heart J* 28:230–268, 2007.

Pibarot P, Dumesnil JG: Prosthetic heart valves: selection of the optimal prosthesis and long-term management, *Circulation* 119:1034–1048, 2009.

Topic 7

Braunwald's Heart Disease: *A textbook of cardiovascular medicine*, ed 7, Elsevier.

Klein AL, Garcia MJ, editors: *Diastology – Clinical Approach to Diastolic Heart Failure*, Elsevier/Saunders.

Troughton RW, Asher CR, Klein AL: Pericarditis, *Lancet* 363:717–727, 2004.

Topic 8

Gatzoulis MA, Swan L, Therrien J, Pantely G, Braunwald E: *Adult Congenital Heart Disease: A Practical Guide*, 2005, Blackwell Publishing.

Management of Grown Up Congenital Heart Disease: The Task Force on the Management of Grown Up Congenital Heart Disease of the European Society of Cardiology, *Eur Heart J* 24:1035–1084, 2003.

Michael HC, John PD, Walter JP: *Cardiology*, 2004, Elsevier.

Thorne S, Clift P, editors: *Adult Congenital Heart Disease. Oxford Specialist Handbooks in Cardiology*, 2009, Oxford University Press.

Warnes CA, Williams RG, Bashore TM, et al: ACC/AHA 2008 Guidelines for the Management of Adults with Congenital Heart Disease, *Circulation* 118:e714–e833, 2008.

Welton MG, Marlon SR: *Congenital Heart Disease in the Adult*, 2002, McGraw-Hill.

Topic 9

British Thoracic Society guidelines for the management of suspected acute pulmonary embolism. British Thoracic Society Standards of Care Committee Pulmonary Embolism Guideline, *Thorax* 58:470–484, 2003.

Galiè N, Torbicki A, Barst R, et al: Guidelines on diagnosis and treatment of pulmonary arterial hypertension. The Task Force on Diagnosis and Treatment of Pulmonary Arterial Hypertension of the European Society of Cardiology, *Eur Heart J* 25:2243–2278, 2004.

The Task Force for the Diagnosis and Treatment of Pulmonary Hypertension of the European Society of Cardiology (ESC) and the European Respiratory Society (ERS), endorsed by the International Society of Heart and Lung Transplantation (ISHLT): Guidelines for the diagnosis and treatment of pulmonary hypertension, *Eur Heart J* 30:2493–2537, 2009.

Topic 10

Li AE, Kamel I, Rando F, et al: Using MRI to assess aortic wall thickness in the multiethnic study of atherosclerosis: distribution by race, sex, and age, *AJR Am J Roentgenol* 182:593–597, 2004.

Appendix 1

British National Formulary: RPS Publishing.

Colucci WS, Elkayam U, Horton DP, et al: Intravenous nesiritide, a natriuretic peptide, in the treatment of decompensated congestive heart failure. Nesiritide Study Group, *N Engl J Med* 343:246–253, 2000.

Hohnloser SH, Crijns HJ, van Eickels M, et al: Effect of dronedarone on cardiovascular events in atrial fibrillation, *NEJM* 360:668–678, 2009.

Mebazaa A, Nieminen MS, Packer M, et al: Levosimendan vs dobutamine for patients with acute decompensated heart failure: The SURVIVE randomized trial, *JAMA* 297:1883–1891, 2007.

Montalescot G, Wiviott SD, Braunwald E, et al: Prasugrel compared with clopidogrel in patients undergoing percutaneous coronary intervention for ST-elevation myocardial infarction (TRITON-TIMI 38): double-blind, randomised controlled trial, *Lancet* 373:723–731, 2009.

Morrow DA, Scirica BM, Karwatowska-Prokopczuk E, et al: Effects of ranolazine on recurrent cardiovascular events in patients with non-ST-elevation acute coronary syndromes: The MERLIN-TIMI 36 randomized trial, *JAMA* 297:1775–1783, 2007.

Tardif JC, Ponikowski P, Kahan T, et al: Efficacy of the If current inhibitor ivabradine in patients with chronic stable angina receiving beta-blocker therapy: a 4-month, randomized, placebo-controlled trial, *Eur Heart J* 30:540–548, 2009.

Appendix 2

United Kingdom Department of Vehicle Licensing and Transport Regulations (Revised November 2008) from Department of Vehicle Licensing Agency.

Index

NB: Page numbers in *italics* refer to figures and tables